A NEW MODEL
FOR HEALTH
AND DISEASE

A NEW MODEL
FOR HEALTH
AND DISEASE

GEORGE VITHOULKAS

Health and Habitat
Mill Valley, California
and
North Atlantic Books
Berkeley, California

ISBN 1-55643-087-6

Published by:
Health and Habitat
76 Lee Street
Mill Valley, CA 94941
and
North Atlantic Books
P.O. Box 12327
Berkeley, CA 94712

Book design and typesetting by Julia Cagwin
Cover design by Paula Morrison
Printed in the United States of America by Malloy Lithographing

A New Model for Health and Disease is sponsored by the Society for the Study of Native Arts and Sciences, a nonprofit educational corporation whose goals are to develop an educational and crosscultural perspective linking various scientific, social, and artistic fields; to nurture a holistic view of the arts, sciences, humanities, and healing; and to publish and distribute literature on the relationship of mind, body, and nature; and by Health and Habitat, a nonprofit educational corporation whose purpose is to promote a holistic approach to life, health, and the environment and to help achieve a healthy healthy state of equilibrium through education, research, homeopathy, conservation of resources, and public charity.

Dedicated to my beloved wife . . .

IN APPRECIATION

I feel obliged first of all to thank the following people whose assistance was invaluable in writing this small treatise:

— Alexandra Delinick, M.D., for her patience and dedication in helping to put my ideas in book form;
— Michael Lefas, M.D., for his invaluable help with the immense research required to support the book's hypotheses;
— George Guess, M.D., my American editor, for his great contributions of time and energy in editing and reviewing this book;
— Sandy Ross, Ph.D., my American assistant, for her devotion and tireless efforts for many years on behalf of all of my work; and her foundation, Health and Habitat, for producing this book and my *Materia Medica Viva*.
— Julia Cagwin, typesetter, of the Wild Flower Press, Mill Valley, California, for her perserverance and guidance.
— Gregory Vlamis, for bringing us Nick Jannes, who generously financed a major portion of this book's production.

I also want to thank John Papadopoulos, Assistant Prof., Dept. of Pharmacology, University of Athens, for his invaluable assistance and criticism, Dr. Francis Treuherz for his editing comments, Harvey Haber for his early work and transcriptions, Jean Barnard, granddaughter of American homeopath William Boericke, M.D., for her early editing, and Linda Johnston, M.D., for her assistance, support and dedication. I thank Peggy Chipkin, R.N., F.N.P., for editing the second edition.

I cannot refrain from giving my deepest appreciation and thanks to all my Teachers whom I was privileged to meet in this life. Strangely enough, none were well known in academic circles nor taught at "recognized" institutions of learning; they insisted on continuing their work in "silence" and anonymity.

CONTENTS

FOREWORD

The book is written with a threefold objective in mind:

1. To show that established medicine has failed in its mission to prevent or cure disease. Instead, it is responsible for a degeneration of health of worldwide dimension due to the excessive use of powerful chemical drugs. Because of this practice, even effective alternative therapeutic systems will take years to reverse or correct the situation.
2. To present a new *Model* of health and disease as a new paradigm for the science of medicine. I hope that by enumerating the various natural laws that govern the phenomena of health and disease it will help to clarify those therapeutic modalities that offer optimal results.
3. To point out that such therapeutic systems exist and are available today, but are either suppressed or intentionally neglected by a large majority of the medical authorities in the world.

The book is primarily addressed to the medical practitioners of the world and the world's authorities, but it has been written in such a manner that a lay person can easily understand.

I must apologize if the reader perceives this book as being written in a polemic or prejudiced manner. I sense a rapidly approaching planetary catastrophe; the style of writing reflects the urgency I feel about this problem. This unfortunate condition has resulted from an unwise and excessive use of prescription and non-prescription drugs and has given rise (according to the author's estimation and research) to the AIDS epidemic, and will probably give rise to worse problems in the future.

It would be wrong if the book were received as only a critique on allopathic medicine. It is because I want the reader's atten-

tion focused on the negative aspects of modern medicine that I
have stressed these points.

Research and inquiry into the deepest recesses of the human
body and mind have revealed extremely interesting aspects
about the makeup of the human being; unfortunately researchers have not perceived the underlying principles of medicine and
health which have always existed as "eternal truths."

I hold special esteem for those dedicated and earnest scientists who have toiled in their laboratories trying to decode and
understand the secrets of nature. I have unlimited admiration
for them because they have passionately dedicated their lives to
the attainment of their scientific goals. But this admiration does
not prevent me from assessing that established medicine has
followed the wrong course of action.

I hope to clearly show in the following pages that the basis of
medical research and therapeutic application has been not only
wrong but also disastrous for the health of mankind.

This book is presented as a hopeful message for a New Era of
Medicine.

The Author
Alonissos, Greece
August 1987

INTRODUCTION

In 1972, while lecturing to a group of medical doctors in Athens, Greece, I made the following statement: "Because of the frequency with which antibiotics are prescribed today by the medical profession, the immune system will soon become weakened to the extent that a host of new, more virulent and incurable diseases will make their appearance. The excessive use of antibiotics deleteriously affects the immune system, in many instances damaging it irreparably."

What prompted the announcement of this gloomy prediction was my own experience in the health field. My statement was quite a controversial one to make in front of physicians, since established medicine considers antibiotics just about the most "astonishing and effective" ammunition they have in combatting disease. But, by 1972 I had already seen and treated hundreds of cases in which I could clearly discern that the appearance of their chronic problems was directly connected to excessive usage of allopathic drugs, usually antibiotics, in particular the penicillin derivatives.

Apart from this specific observation, I was aware, like others in the health field, that there was a general degeneration of health taking place in that part of the world which boasted of having the best and most expensive medical care. We see this degeneration evident in the life expectancy of males in the United States. Compared with other developed nations (all of which spend substantially less for health care) the United States ranks nineteenth in mortality rates.[1]

It is obvious from the following statistics that there are many developing countries in South America where life expectancy is longer than in the U.S. If, in fact, the most expensive and best medical care is responsible for the longest life expectancy, then the U.S. should have that honor; but in actuality, the opposite is true.

1

We present the life expectancies for males in a cross-section of countries in North, Central and South America:

	1981	1982	1983	1984	1985
Costa Rica:	—	—	74.5	—	—
Puerto Rico:	70.8	73.2	—	—	—
Panama:	—	72.8	72.9	—	—
Barbados:	—	—	—	72.0	—
Cuba:	—	—	—	72.2	—

In the United States it was only 70.1 years in 1980, 70.5 in 1981, 70.9 in 1982, and 71 in 1983.[2,3,4]

We can come to the same conclusions in Europe, where Greece and Iceland, two of the still-developing countries, possess the best life expectancy and mortality rates. In the Eastern bloc countries we see the figures are quite low, with Hungary leading the way. Of the industrialized nations of Europe, Sweden has the best life expectancy rate, and then, in decreasing order, we have the Netherlands, Norway, England and Wales, France, Fed. Rep. of Germany, Italy, Belgium and finally, Austria with the worst rate.[2,3,4]

	1981	1982	1983	1984	1985
Iceland:	—	74.7	—	74.9	—
Greece:	—	73.6	—	73.8	—
Sweden:	73.1	—	—	73.9	—
Austria:	—	69.4	—	—	70.4
Hungary:	—	65.6	—	65.1	—

Eastern bloc countries, in spite of supposedly complete medical coverage and forced immunization of the whole population, post the lowest life expectancies. I hope to make clear with the theory I shall present that this phenomenon is no paradox.[2,3,4]

	1981	1982	1983	1984	1985
Hungary:	—	65.6	—	65.1	65.1
Czechoslovakia:	67.0	—	66.9	67.1	—
Romania:	—	67.1	66.9	67.1	—
Poland:	67.1	67.3	67.1	66.8	—
Bulgaria:	—	68.5	68.3	68.5	—

Thus, we see that the plain numbers tell a story different from the one usually given by the medical establishment. It usually says that the life expectancy has risen because of better medical care. Besides that, the above data give us a picture of only the quantitative side of the issue, without touching upon the **quality** of life offered by modern medicine.

What is the quality of life for those living on kidney dialysis or with heart transplants, epilepsy, rheumatoid arthritis, Alzheimer's disease, cancer or AIDS? All these people are included in the statistics evaluating life expectancy, yet the quality of their lives may well be such as to throw the value of a long life, per se, in doubt. Quality of life—the amount of joy, happiness and creativity that gives purpose to our lives—must be considered in addition to life's duration before any meaningful conclusions can be reached about the effects of any health care plan.

How many of us live in such a healthy state that we can really enjoy life and be creative at the same time? To measure the degree of health which a population enjoys is a difficult and arduous task, especially when one is dealing with statistics; but it is something that, some day, has to be done one way or another. I can even predict that if we carry on in the same manner as in the past, we shall very soon be witnessing a drop even in the quantitative statistics of developed countries. If we had the ability or the will to measure our quality of health, I am sure that we would change our medical system immediately.

Since nobody is doing such an evaluation, we are forced to rely on our own perceptions and experiences in order to answer pertinent questions like:

— How satisfied are you with the drugs you've been receiving for your different chronic ailments?

— In the long run, based on your own experience, are these drugs causing you harm in other levels of your health?

— How has the quality of your life been affected by such drugs?

— Even though you may no longer be experiencing disturbing symptoms, do you feel that your health is really back to normal?

— How do you feel about constantly taking tranquilizers, sedatives, painkillers, bronchodilators, hormonal products, cortisone and other drugs?

— Is our medical system really a curative one, or one that just manages to "suppress" disease symptoms?

What we place into our body affects every level of our being. The quantity and quality of the different drugs that go into our body play a great part in upgrading or downgrading the **quality** of our existence, which really is what life is all about.

In the last fifteen years we have constantly witnessed the appearance of new diseases. Between 1972 and 1980 some fifteen "new" diseases made their appearance. Their causes were unknown, puzzling and elusive. How responsible for this phenomenon were the chemical drugs we were then using? Is it possible that there is a connection between the phenomenon of drug "overuse" and the inability of our immune systems to prevent the appearance of these alarming new diseases?

In addition to the appearance of new diseases, there is also an outbreak of fungal infections. By 1975 I was already witnessing an increasing number of patients suffering from such infections. Lately we are witnessing such a tremendous "explosion" of dermal and genital mycoses that this phenomenon is close to becoming a universal problem. In Great Britain the new cases of candida alone, due to the fungus *Candida Albicans,* increased from 34,696 in 1973 to 64,173 in 1984.[5] In Britain, it was ranked second among all venereal diseases in 1984.[6] Quite a number of authorities attribute much of today's "chronic systemic symptomatology" to fungi. Raymond Keith in his book *AIDS, Cancer and the Medical Establishment* states that, "In recent years, chronic and often imperceptible Candida infections have been recognized as associated with severe symptoms referable **to every system of the body**."[7]

I stopped to think what could have caused this tremendous rise in fungal infections, and then I realized that one of the major antibiotics prescribed to millions by medical doctors was nothing but a **fungus** derivative, a mold! The common name of this mold is **penicillin**. In effect, thousands of tons of this drug have been pumped into human organisms since the second World War. There is hardly anybody left in the developed countries who has escaped this "wonder drug." Just to give you a general idea of the amounts of antibiotics consumed, we quote some figures: in the U.S. alone, the annual production of antibiotics in the year 1965 was 7.3 million pounds, but by 1970 it was 16.9 million pounds. Within four years, between 1967 and 1971, the number of prescriptions for ampicillin alone increased from 9.5

million to 21.5 million.[8] The Food and Drug Administration's (FDA) antibiotic certification records show that the volume of injectable cephalosporins and gentamycin administered has increased steadily and as of 1977 was still rising.[9]

In order to combat infections, the required dosage of antibiotics has risen tremendously due to the fact that organisms have become less and less susceptible to them. To give you an example of the increasing dosages of penicillin necessary to combat infections such as gonorrhea, dosage requirements are cited from old pharmacology texts, as well as from Goodman and Gilman's *Pharmaceutical Basis of Therapeutics,* 5th ed., 1985:

"When gonorrhea was first treated with procaine penicillin the treatment required a few hundred thousands of units (300,000 IU). But as the human system developed more and more resistance to it, the amount increased to millions of units (4,800,000 IU penicillin + 1g probenecid)." This is **sixteenfold the initial amount.**

It was obvious that penicillin, a fungus derivative, was more powerful than microbes and bacteria in the body, because once inserted in the organism it would immobilize them.[10] But in this way **penicillin (a fungus)** was insidiously establishing its **own reign** in the body, and it appeared that it was there to stay for good.

Then, more and more powerful drugs were developed, e.g. amphotericin-B, flucytosine, ketoconazole, miconazole, to combat the steadily increasing lethal power of fungi. But at what cost? According to Dr. H. Simmons:

"Iatrogenic disease in the U.S. has become a serious public health problem. This includes an estimated two million nosocomial infections and many thousands of deaths per year. As others have already pointed out, a substantial amount of this is attributable to the inappropriate use of anti-infective agents."[10]

Soon different voices from within the medical profession started raising their objections, but unfortunately, nobody took notice.

"The real tragedy lies in the fact that infectious-disease experts have been pointing out these problems and desperately crying out for change for the past thirty years—largely to no avail."[10]

Some hard questions were raised in an editorial published in the *Journal of the American Medical Association,* entitled "This is Medical Progress?"[8] These questions were:

" —Has the wide use of antibiotics led to the emergence of new resistant bacterial strains?
— Has the ecology of 'natural' or 'hospital' bacterial flora been shifted because of antibiotic use?
— Have nosocomial infections changed in incidence or severity due to antibiotic use?
— What are the trends of antibiotic use?
— Is the increasingly more frequent use of antibiotics presenting the medical community and the public with a new set of hazards that should be approached by some new administrative or educational measures?
— Are antibiotics properly used in practice?"

and it continues:

"Along with the dramatic decline in the rates of formerly lethal diseases, **new and major** hazards have also emerged, due to antibiotic therapy." [8]

This, like many others, was an early warning of the hazards of medication. What the warning was about was that although the new "wonder drugs" decreased deaths from acute infectious diseases, they added a new dimension to the manifestation and propagation of chronic diseases. As Rene Dubos so appropriately states in his book *So Human an Animal:*

"While they have done much in the prevention and treatment of a few specific diseases, they have so far failed to increase true longevity or to create positive health. The age of affluence, technological marvels, and medical miracles is paradoxically the age of chronic ailments, of anxiety, and even of despair."

Also, because the over-utilization of antimicrobial agents has precipitated the emergence of more virulent infectious organisms, the management of acute infectious diseases has, in general, become more difficult.

Today, thirteen years later, in spite of this information, even stronger drugs are in use by the medical profession.

It is only logical that now, after all these facts have surfaced, certain questions arise concerning the widespread use of antibiotics and their effect upon the human body.

1. Is there a possibility that penicillin and its derivatives have caused changes or faults in the immune system such that it can no longer resist the colonization of the body by different species of fungi?

Here are some reports from different investigators who respond to this question:

Fungi have emerged as major pathogens, especially in immunosuppressed patients who have prolonged granulocytopenia and protracted courses of antibiotic therapy.[11]

Suppression of T-cell function by tetracycline could partially explain the superinfection by Candida sometimes seen clinically after prolonged use of these agents.[12]

Immunomodulation (deficiency of the immune system) must be added to the myriad of potential antibiotic side effects.[14]

For more specific information we cite references: [13,15,16,17]

2. Is it possible that the irresponsible use of these drugs, and thus the resultant mutation of microorganisms, is preparing the way for the manifestation of some dreadful, incurable diseases with new and unrecognizable mutants (new viruses, fungi, etc.)?

Several sources are cited with statistical data that give an ample answer to the above questions:

"Infections caused by Gram-negative bacilli are becoming increasingly prevalent and currently constitute the most frequent type of nosocomial infection. Several major centers have reported an annual frequency of Gram-negative bacteremia of approximately 1 per 100 hospital patients, with fatality rates of 30% - 50%. If similar incidence and fatality rates hold for the 30,000,000 acute hospital admissions annually in the United States, as many as 300,000 episodes and more than 100,000 fatalities from Gram-negative bacteremia may occur each year." [8]

"In one study, using strict criteria, a superinfection rate of 2.2% was noted in more than 3,000 patients treated with antibiotics. The most striking fact about this study was that Gram-negative bacteria were involved in the majority of these 'superinfections' and they were much more difficult to manage than the primary disorder." [18]

Because of the irresponsible way in which antibiotics generally are prescribed to the public we have the "continuing emergence of even more dangerous and resistant bacterial strains with which the next generation of antibiotics must try to cope."[10]

It has been cited in the literature that antibiotics "may have marked effects on host-parasite interactions" in the form of producing multiple drug resistance by actually inducing certain mutations to occur, by the production of alterations on their surface structure due to their adaptation to the selective pressure of the antibiotics.[19]

Thus "originally sensitive bacteria may develop drug resistance through mutation, plasmids, or may acquire it by one of the processes necessitating transfer of genetic material from resistant to sensitive organisms." [20]

Also several other mechanisms are cited such as alterations of the bacterial chromosomes, enzymatic inactivation of the antibiotics, and establishment of a drug permeability barrier.[21]

We have multiple cases where newer and stronger strains of microorganisms developed that were less drug-sensitive and more drug-resistant. One case involved a neurosurgical unit where infections by Klebsiella aerogenes had reached epidemic proportions because "ampicillin and cloxacillin had been used for years as 'prophylaxis.' "[20]

In previously mentioning the transfer of genetic material in inducing drug resistance, we have the example of the R-factor. R-factors have "been identified in high incidence among hospital strains of Pseudomonas aeruginosa." These R-factors, which determine **multiple resistance**, can be easily transmitted from one strain of Pseudomonas aeruginosa to another, therefore making it harder for even the "aminoglycoside antibiotics" to deal with them.[22] So these bacteria have actually been made **stronger** by the same "antibiotics" that were intended to destroy them.

Another antibiotic-induced resistance is the "emergence of the resistance to ... the newer B-lactam antibiotics."[23]

"Since the introduction of penicillin forty years ago, penicillin resistance has increased in staphylococci and now at least 80% of staphylococci from developed countries produce B-lactamase."[24] B-lactamase is the substance that makes the staphylococcus resistant to penicillin. Also, "particular resistance to penicillin has become an increasing problem in the control of gonorrhea."[25]

"Methicillin-resistant staphylococcus aureus has emerged as a nationwide problem in some U.S. hospitals. Staphylococcus aureus infections began sweeping U.S. hospitals in the late 1970s and reached epidemic proportion by the early 1980s."[26]

"The rapidity with which different resistance genes, transposons and R plasmids have spread to various pathogens around the world demonstrates the powerful selective forces imposed by human use of antibiotics. However, a recent survey of over 400 enterobacteria collected and subsequently stored between 1917 and 1954 suggests that resistance was very uncommon in the pre-antibiotic era... The ultimate sources of many resistance genes are likely to be the soil microorganisms that actually produce most antibiotics or that would be competing with such producers. Since antibiotics are potentially toxic to the producing organism, it is hardly surprising that bacteria such as streptomycetes should possess resistance mechanisms to protect themselves from the antibiotics they produce."[27]

Some scientists and medical researchers truly believe that we may be returning to a **"pre-antibiotic era in which these transformed multiresistant microorganisms will again devastate mankind.** This alarm is due to the observed selective pressure in both human and nonhuman microbial environments exerted by the widespread and ever-increasing use of antibiotics."[27]

Perhaps it has not been understood so far, that the quality of our health depends almost entirely on the quality of microorganisms that exist normally within our body and thus form the basis of our life. If we disturb their equilibrium by pumping all this "mold" into the organism, we are going to have a "moldy" organism eventually.

It has been stated that the "prescribing of antibiotics, whether inside or outside hospitals, adds needlessly to the mounting pressures for selection of resistant organisms. It may seem an overstatement to describe it as an act of environmental pollution, but when the full and ultimate consequences of this manner of use are grasped it is less of an exaggeration than might have at first appeared."[20]

So far, it seems that modern medicine has not been concerned with the vital issue of the quality of microorganisms that live normally within the body and the mutation these microorganisms are undergoing because of the influence of foreign substances like antibiotics. **The outcome has been a transformation, a mutation, from which a non-pathogenic bacteria is turned into a pathogenic one**; e.g. Alcaligenes, a non-pathogenic bacteria, which exists normally in the human microflora and is an antibiotic-resistant organism, may transfer its resistance to **previous non-resistant** but potentially lethal organisms, such as Pseudomonas aerigunosa.[22]

Transferable drug resistance, which means antibiotic resistance that can be transferred from one species of bacteria to another, though first demonstrated only in intestinal bacteria, has become commonplace in many other bacteria as well.[28-34]

In effect, the widespread use of antibiotics has created on all levels of the organism a hazardous situation that is now very difficult to either undo or correct.

3. Is it possible that all developed countries and some in the process of developing have been using extremely powerful drugs in an extremely unwise way? Was it possible that apart from the damage that came as a necessary evil to life-threatening situations, there

were other instances where these powerful agents were used indiscriminately?

The evidence for such practices is overwhelming, as you can see from the following quotations:

When a physician prescribes a medication for a patient, the act is often shaped, in a large part, by forces unrelated to the biochemical properties of the drug—a phenomenon which has been called "the non-pharmacological basis of therapeutics".[35]

For more information on this please note references.[36-43]

"In 1968 the Health, Education and Welfare (HEW) Task Force on Prescription Drugs devised this definition, and expressed the conclusion that rational prescribing as so defined was far from universal in medical practice... 'It is my belief,' said Dr. Jan Koch-Weser of Harvard, 'that lack of knowledge in the proper therapeutic use of drugs is perhaps the greatest deficiency of the average American physician today.' " [44]

"Prescription surveys give some idea of the extent of inappropriate drug use. For example: Of the 25 most frequently prescribed drugs in the U.S. in 1976, eight were authoritatively considered to be pharmacologically or therapeutically questionable. (Knapp D.E., 1978; cited in Smith M.C., 1980)...An analysis of over 50,000 teaching hospital prescriptions in the U.S. indicated a higher than 1 in 8 level of over-medication (excessive quantities of drugs and/or frequency of dosage). There was also a significant number of inappropriate combinations of drugs (risk of reduced therapeutic effect and/or harmful drug interaction). (Maronde et al., 1971) ...The list of studies showing inadequate practice is extensive and they are not limited to office practice. Hendeles (1976) cited two hospital studies which discovered inappropriate use of antibiotics in over 60% of cases (Smith M.C., 1980). A later study of prescribing in Scottish hospitals supports these findings: 'In two-thirds of such patients, there was no good bacteriological evidence that an antibiotic was required. Since 11% of all antibiotic exposures were associated with undesirable side effects, it was concluded that the risks of therapy were greater than the benefit to be expected' " (Moir D., et al., 1979).[45]

A retrospective analysis of randomly selected patients, according to the Kunin's categories of use, showed 64% of the total antibiotic therapy as not indicated or inappropriately administered in terms of drug or dosage.[46]

"In 50.5% of hospital discharges in 1972 where antibiotics were given, no record of a bacterial culture was recorded on the chart."[8]

The striking production figures for the tetracyclines are somewhat surprising in view of the warnings about using tetracyclines in children or infants.[47]

"—Lack of understanding by many physicians as to the proper use of anti-infective agents and their pharmacological properties,

— Widespread use of anti-infective agents in conditions for which they are either known to be ineffective, or where there is a lack of substantial evidence of efficacy,

— Overextensive and inappropriate use of powerful or broad-spectrum antibiotics in instances where simpler, safer or less expensive, or no antibiotic, therapy would suffice,

— Significant deficiencies in knowledge among physicians of the proper use of bacteriological laboratory and interpretation of the findings.

These factors combine to lead to substantial harm, significant waste, serious ethical questions of prolongation of many already severely compromised lives..." [10]

4. Is it possible that drugs have been used in human organisms without being properly tested for long-term effects?

The most classical examples of adverse long-term effects from drugs that were supposed to have been tested properly are:

— Thalidomide, which circulated in the 1950s as a tranquilizer and produced the well known genetic defect known as phocomelia.

— Phenylbutazone, an anti-inflammatory drug which produces suppression of the bone marrow. In 1983, the fact that 1200 deaths were attributed to this drug was kept quiet. The drug is still in use although there is no apparent need for it, according to the World Health Organization (WHO).

— Indoprophene, an anti-inflammatory drug taken off the market in 1985 because of certain allusions to the drug's carcinogenesis.

— Clioquinol, an anti-diarrhetic drug: On the record in Japan alone, there were 11,000 disability cases and 1,000 deaths. The major adverse effect was that it caused SMON (Syndrome of Myelo-Optic Neuropathy).

— Phenacetin, an analgesic that produces renal insufficiency. [47]

The Food and Drug Administration (FDA) investigations turned up various sorry aspects of what was touted as research: the submission of detailed reports and claims involving a series of two patients **only**; claims of therapeutic miracles on patients who had not even been adequately diagnosed; the use of private physicians as drug company experts who were delighted—at a price—to sign any endorsement, provided that somebody would tell them what to report. As one reporter noted:

"Some drug companies went so far as to design the 'clinical' experiment, write the testing physician's reports, and then pay him for use of his name." [44]

"During the past few years it has been reported that cancer of the vagina—ordinarily an exceedingly rare type of malignancy—has been detected in almost a hundred young girls whose mothers had been given stilbestrol to prevent an apparently imminent spontaneous abortion. The first use of the drug for this purpose dates back to 1946. In 1953 two controlled trials demonstrated its complete lack of efficacy. Yet the director of the Clinical Center of the National Institute of Health testified that in the late 1940s, 1950s and 1960s, without proof of benefit, thousands of pregnant women underwent stilbestrol therapy." [44]

"The increase in the use of drugs for both short-term and long-term treatment during the past decades has led to a corresponding increase in concern about their potential for inducing serious illnesses (illnesses that are potentially life-threatening or otherwise produce substantial incapacity, disability or both)." [48]

But the most alarming report comes from John Braithwaite, where in his well-researched book *Corporate Crime of the Pharmaceutical Industry*, he describes the unethical way that certain drugs were tested. On page 51 he writes:

"Dr. Ley, Goddard's immediate successor at the helm of the Food and Drug Administration (FDA), told hearings before the U.S. Senate…of one spot check which turned up the case of an assistant professor of medicine who had reputedly tested twenty-four drugs for nine different companies. 'Patients who died while on clinical trials were not reported to the sponsor,' an audit revealed. Dead people were listed as subjects of testing. People reported as subjects of testing were not in the hospital at the time of the tests. Patient consent forms bore dates indicating they were signed by the subjects after the subjects died." He reports further that in studies conducted by one commercial drug-testing firm, "Patients who died, left the hospital or dropped out of the study were replaced by other patients in the tests without notification in the records. Forty-one patients reported as participants in studies were dead or not in the hospital during the study…." [49]

Of course, I do not mean to imply that all pharmaceutical companies follow the same unethical practices, but the fact remains that the consequences of allopathic drugs are too often tragic or disastrous for quite a number of people. What is even more grim is the fact that nobody today can predict the subtle long-term effects that chemical drugs may have upon the human organism. Additional literature describing adverse symptoms or side effects can be found in abundance in medical journals cited in references.[50-54] Several researchers have reported an alarming ignorance on the part of physicians concerning the use of antibiotics.[55,56,57]

For the last fifteen years I have been trying to draw the attention of the medical profession to these really deadly issues. I have spoken at different universities in America and in Europe—always as a guest of the medical students. I have spoken passionately in my yearly seminars to physicians all over the world about these issues, and nobody seems to argue with me about the validity of these assumptions. Concerning a talk I gave in San Francisco in 1978, Richard Grossinger wrote:

"When Vithoulkas spoke at the University of California Hospital in San Francisco, he received a five-minute standing ovation from the medical personnel, despite the fact that he had demolished in his lecture everything that the medicine practiced in that building stood for."[58]

In essence, most people agree on the validity of these statements, yet there has been no change forthcoming. Many authorities have issued similar warnings over the years, but there has been no change in the medical way of thinking. Perhaps what is needed now is for medical centers to consider these thoughts, investigate these matters and publish their own conclusions. There is already enough scientific evidence to support the claims presented here. However, if these institutions need more research, they should perform it quickly. A tempest of maladies is rapidly approaching, and it is not going to spare anyone.

At the end of this book, I advance a hypothesis which states that the AIDS situation is very much connected to the **occurrence and treatment** of venereal disease. Some of my ideas relating to this issue are pertinent to the topic here under discussion.

In the beginning, it was apparent to me and to many venerologists that "non-specific urethritis" was nothing else but the continuation of the gonorrheal infection in a more latent and chronic form. Often-repeated prescriptions of antibiotics did nothing to alleviate the condition. While gonorrhea seemed to be decreasing, in reality the gonorrheal affliction, under the pressure of antibiotics, was being transformed into non-specific urethritis or ascending urinary infections. In fact, non-specific urethritis is approaching epidemic proportions in the population. Several authorities have referred to this matter.

This is also evident in that there is a "continued increase in annual incidence of **non-gonococcal urethritis (NGU)** at a time when gonorrhea is coming under control in some western countries," underscoring "the need to examine critically the epidemiology of NGU." [59]

"Chronic prostatitis may follow gonococcal or non-gonococcal urethritis and is especially common after the latter. Indeed such silent 'prostatitis' almost invariably accompanies non-gonococcal urethritis. Treatment in the absence of a known cause is empirical and often unsatisfactory." [60]

The fact was that we were not really curing the infection but rather "transforming" it into another more chronic form. Researchers attest to the fact that "chronic urethritis infection may represent the end stage of an incompletely healed acute urethritis." [61]

While in previous decades the problem of venereal diseases appeared primarily in the form of syphilis and gonorrhea, in our modern society these two infectious diseases have been relegated to secondary positions. A host of new sexually transmitted diseases has appeared in epidemic proportion in their stead. Such diseases are non-specific genital and urinary infections,

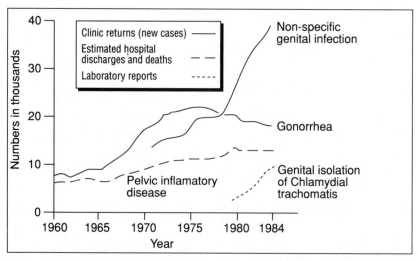

Figure 1: Genital tract infections in women in England and Wales (1960-1984). Epidemiology of Genital Chlamydial Infections; *Infection-1982, 10 (Supp.): S33.*

mainly due to *Chlamydia trachomatis, Candida albicans* (causes candidiasis), the herpes virus (simplex and complex types) and genital wart viruses. (See *Figure 1* and *Figure 2*)

From looking at these first two figures we can come to certain conclusions:

a. It took several years of antibiotic treatment for us to clearly see the long-term side-effects of antibiotics and the extreme rise in non-specific genital infections.
b. In spite of the wide use of broad-spectrum antibiotics, we observe continuing incidence of gonorrhea and a tremendous rise in non-specific genital infections.
c. All of the cases of gonorrhea thought to be cured are now appearing as chronic cases of non-specific genital infections.

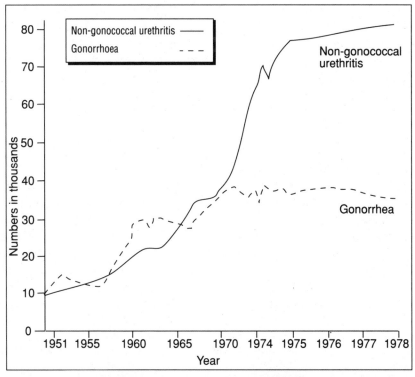

Figure 2: Reported cases of non-gonococcal urethritis and gonorrhea in England and Wales (1951-1978). Sexually transmitted disease surveillance in Britain, 1984; *British Medical Journal-1986, 293: 943.*

Here we have *Chlamydia trachomatis* being "responsible for about 50% of **non-specific genital infections.**" (Chlamydial infections are probably the most prevalent of the sexually transmitted diseases.) [62]

The "FDA states flatly that chlamydial infections are 'more prevalent in the United States than any other venereal disease; there are at least three cases for every two of gonorrhea.' ... Three million Americans a year are infected with the chlamydia." [63]

Thus we see that "non-specific genital infections rank first among all sexually transmitted diseases." [5.6]

According to my hypothesis, what was actually taking place in all gonorrhea treatment with antibiotics was that the infection, when treated repeatedly with these drugs, was pushed deeper into the organism, resulting in chronic inflammation of the prostate gland or ascending urinary and genital infections.

The following statements lend this hypothesis validity:

"Chronic prostatitis usually develops as a result of invasion of bacteria from the urethra"; [61] "gonococcal prostatitis occurs only in men who have had prior histories of gonococcal urethritis." [64]

"Chronic non-bacterial prostatitis is much more common than chronic bacterial prostatitis. It is an ill-understood condition which shows a poor response to therapy. Most patients had had one or more courses of antimicrobials before they were referred for prostatic investigation. This (treatment) may be sufficient to prevent the culture of microorganisms but insufficient to **suppress** [emphasis mine] symptoms or prevent predisposition to recurrent non-specific urethritis." [65]

When medical doctors talk about suppressing the symptoms they do not realize that what they necessarily imply is that another condition representing the symptom on a deeper level will most probably manifest. Medical education has not yet sensitized physicians to the fact that they should be viewing the human being as a whole and not a mere collection of parts. So they are not aware that in suppressing a symptom they may actually be causing harm to the whole organism.

"Both acute and chronic bacterial prostatitis can be associated with reinfections of the urethra when patients are followed for several years after obtaining bacteriological cures." [66]

"Early observations of patients with chronic bacterial prostatitis revealed that sensitive bacteria persisted in the prostatic fluid despite the serum levels of bactericidal drugs that far exceeded the minimal inhibitory concentration of the infecting organism." [67] What this means is that pathological organisms persist in the prostatic fluid, in spite of huge doses of antibiotics. [68]

Thus we see that when a specific urethritis was thwarted with antibiotics, either a non-specific urethritis, a prostatitis or a genital infection appeared.

As a consequence, I was not surprised to see that in 1981 a new virus was traced which was found mostly in 'promiscuous' homosexual males. The common denominator between my theory and the discovery of the virus is that in this particular group, syphilis or gonorrheal infections are quite frequent and are treated with antibiotics. Many of these homosexuals also use antibiotics prophylactically before casual sexual encounters, thus increasing their antibiotic use 50- to 100-fold as compared to the rest of the population.

— Is it therefore possible that treatment with these drugs, combined with the specific stress on the organism induced by the venereal disease, could lead to the immune system's depleted state and thus allow the development of the "new virus" ?

— Is it possible that the "deficiency" was "acquired" primarily because of the preceding antibiotic treatments?

— How is it possible that the previously strong immune systems of young male homosexuals could be destroyed within a few years of their beginning their homosexual practices?

— Can we accuse male homosexuality for the AIDS disease? This question has been asked and researched by very serious researchers.

These are questions that I shall attempt to answer in the following chapters. But I would like to repeat that before one can fully understand my theory on AIDS, one will have to read the entire book in order that all elements of my argument may be appreciated.

The ideas I am proposing in this *Model* are not the theoretical whims of my imagination, but principles that have been formulated from 28 years of experience and observations in treating more than 150,000 patients with a great variety of diseases. The overall supervision and observation of such a large number of cases was possible because I was the director of a large clinic in Athens, Greece, where thirty medical doctors were practicing an alternative therapeutic discipline.

It is also important that the reader not lose sight of the objectives set forth by this *Model* which are:

1. To formulate the basic laws and principles that govern the human body in health and disease.
2. To explain the reason or reasons for the human race's present degenerated state of health.
3. To help the reader decide which is the best way to treat human disease.
4. To help the reader realize that in transgressing the existing laws of nature, consequences must be borne.

I would like to reiterate that I do not blame or hold responsible the individual scientists, corporations, pharmaceutical companies, universities or governments for the current state of affairs pertaining to our "health." I do believe that all those concerned with health issues have worked earnestly and conscientiously, according to their understanding and abilities, to provide the best health care they thought possible. But I also believe that the majority of them have been caught up in a vicious circle of "apparent truths" which resulted from asking the wrong questions and obstinately pursuing elusive answers. The end result has been chaos. In general, my belief is that medical research has taken the wrong direction.

The question usually asked in research laboratories is : **"Can we find a chemical or biological substance that will eliminate the pathological agent?"**

It may sound paradoxical, but this is the **wrong question** to ask. This question and others similarly misguided have led research efforts astray. These efforts have been directed toward finding agents which could "kill" viruses, bacteria or fungi. In reality what has been happening is that once a chemical has been inserted into the body, it not only destroys the harmful bacteria, but also other useful microorganisms which are absolutely necessary to maintain the body's homeostasis.

Perhaps the right questions are:

1. Why does the organism allow a disease state to occur in the first place?
2. How can we best support the body's natural defenses so that it can rid itself of the disease?

3. Is there any way available to restore health other than to kill the pathological agents with chemical drugs?

I consider it **vital** that these questions should have been asked from the very beginning by those engaged in medical research; but nobody has thus far seemed concerned with such deliberations.

No one denies the fact that so far research has been conducted with integrity and the best of intentions. Without wishing to denigrate their integrity or good intentions, however, it is time that I reveal my evidence and offer my observations of the natural principles governing health and disease.

Because of past "scientific" conditioning, the new ideas contained in *A New Model for Health and Disease* initially may appear abstract, advanced and perhaps foreign to the reader; but as we are dealing with new material and ideas, I ask the reader to be patient and not pass judgment until he or she has read the whole treatise.

I would also like to state from the beginning that this thesis about a **new *Model* of health and disease** is only an hypothesis which attempts to give insight into the human being's mode of functioning during health and disease and into the construction of the human being in all its levels of existence. The main effort will be to provide a theoretical *Model* that will explain the "manifestation" of disease and the tremendous increase of chronic degenerative illnesses in our time.

I also feel obliged to state that the task I have undertaken is tremendously difficult and extremely complicated, and thus my attempt is by no means complete or final. It is only a suggestion of the direction toward which medical thinking should proceed in order to free itself from the vicious circle in which it is now entangled.

REFERENCES:

1. McKINLAY JB, McKINLAY SM: The questionable contribution of medical measures to the decline of mortality in the United States in the twentieth century. *Milbank Mem Fund Q 1977; 55: 405-428*
2. World Health Statistics Annual, *1983*
3. World Health Statistics Annual, *1985*
4. World Health Statistics Annual, *1986*

5. Communicable Disease Surveillance Centre: Sexually transmitted diseases surveillance in Britain: 1983. *Brit Med J 1985; 291: 528-529*

6. Communicable Disease Surveillance Centre: Sexually transmitted diseases surveillance in Britain: 1984. *Brit Med J 1986; 293: 942-943*

7. GOLDBERG PK, KOZZIN PJ, WISE GJ, NOURI N, BROOKS RB: Incidence and significance of candiduria. *JAMA 1979; 241: 582-584*

8. Commentary: This is medical progress? *JAMA 1974; 227: 1023-1028*

9. FINKEL MJ: Magnitude of antibiotic use. *Ann Int Med 1978; 89 (part 2): 791-792*

10. SIMMONS, HE: An overview of public policy and infectious diseases. *Ann Int Med 1978; 89 (part 2): 821-825*

11. PIZZO PA, YOUNG LS: Limitations of current antimicrobial therapy in the immunosuppresed host: looking at both sides of the coin. *Amer J Med 1984; 101-107*

12. MUNSTER AM, BOYD LOADHOLT C, LEARY AG, BARNES MA: The effect of antibiotics on cell-mediated immunity. *Surgery 1977; 81: 692-695*

13. WEISERGER AS, DANIEL TM, HOFFMAN A: Suppression of antibody synthesis and prolongation of homograft survival by chloramphenicol. *J Exp Med 1964; 120: 183*

14. HAUSER WE, REMINGTON JS: Effect of antibiotics on the immune response, *Amer J Med 1982; 72: 711-716*

15. GHILCHIK MW, MORRIS AS, REEVES DS: Immunosuppressive powers of the antimicrobial agent trimethoprim. *Nature 1970; 227: 393-394*

16. GAYLARDE PM, SARCANY I: Suppression of thymidine uptake of human lymphocytes by co-trimoxazole. *Br Med J 1978; 3: 144-146*

17. MUNSTER AM, LOADHOLT CB, LEARY AG, BARNES MA: The effect of antibiotic on cell-mediated immunity. *Surgery 1977; 81: 692-695*

18. WEINSTEIN L, MUSHER DM: Antibiotic induced superinfection. *J Infect Dis 1969; 119: 662-665*

19. STOLLERMAN GH: Trends in bacterial virulence and antibiotic susceptibility: streptococci, pneumonococci and gonococci. *Ann Int Med 1978; 89 (part 2): 746-748*

20. WHITEHEAD JEM: Bacterial resistance: changing patterns of some common pathogens. *Brit Med J 1973; 2: 224-228*

21. BENVISTE R, DAVIES J: Mechanisms of antibiotic resistance in bacteria. *Ann Rev Biochem 1973; 42: 471*

22. HUMMEL RP et al: Antibiotic resistance transfer from nonpathogenic to pathogenic bacteria. *Surgery 1977; 82,3: 382-385*

23. SANDERS CC, SANDERS WE: Microbial resistance to newer generation B-lactam antibiotics: clinical and laboratory implications. *J Infect Dis 1985; 151,3: 399-404*

24. LACEY RW: Antibiotic resistance in Staphylococcus Aureus and Streptococci. *Brit Med Bull 1984; 40,1: 77-83*

25. PLATT DJ: Prevalence of multiple antibiotic resistance in Neisseria Gonorrheae. *Brit J Vener Dis 1976; 52: 384-386*

26. HALEY RW et al: The emergence of methicillin-resistant Staphylococcus aureus infections in United States Hospitals. *Ann Int Med 1982; 97, 3: 297-303*

27. SAUNDERS JR: Genetics and evolution of antibiotic resistance. *Brit Med Bull 1984; 40: 1*

28. McCABE WR, JACKSON GG: Gram-negative bacteremia: Etiology and Ecology. *Arch Int Med 1962; 110: 847-855*

29. EISENSTEIN BI, SOX T, BISWAS G, BLACKMAN E, SRARLING PF: Conjugal transfer of the gonococcal penillicinase plasmid. *Science 1977; 195: 998-1000*

30. KORFHAGEN TR, LOPER JC, FERREL JA: Psedomonas aeruginosa R factors determining gentamicin plus carbenicillin resistance from patients with urinary tract colonizations. *Antimicrob Agents Chemother 1974; 6: 492*

31. MINSHEW BH, HOLMES RK, SANFORD JP: Transferable resistance to tobramycin in Klesbiella pneumonia and enterobacter cloacae associated with enzymatic acetylation of tobramycin. *Antimicrob Agents Chemother 1974; 6: 492*

32. LACEY RW, CHOPRA I: Genetic studies on a multi-resistant strain of staphylococcus aureus. *J Med Microbiol 1974; 7: 285-297*

33. ANDRESON ES: The ecology of transferable drug resistance in the enterobacteria. *Ann Rev Microbiol 1968; 22: 131-180*

34. PANIKERN CK, VIMALA KN: Transferable chloramphenicol resistance in Salmonella typhi. *Nature 1972; 239: 109-112*

35. AVORN J, CHEN M, HARTLEY R: Scientific versus commercial sources of influence on the prescribing behavior of physicians. *Amer J Med 1982; 73: 4-8*

36. MAZZULLO J: The non pharmacological basis of therapeutics. *Clin Pharmacol Ther 1972; 13: 157-158*

37. STOLLEY PD, LASAGNA L: Prescribing patterns of physicians. *J Chronic Dis 1969; 22: 395-405*

38. MILLER RR: Prescribing habits of physicians. *Drug Intell Clin Pharm 1974; 8: 85*

39. HEMMINKI E: Review of literature on the factors affecting drug prescribing. *Soc Sci Med 1975; 9: 111-115*

40. CLUFF L: The prescribing habits of physicians. *Hosp Pract 1967; 101-104*

41. LIEFF J, AVORN JL, CADDELL W, et al: Attitudes of the medical profession toward drug abuse. *Amer J Pubic Health 1973; 63: 1035-1039*

42. AVORN J, SOUMERAI S: De-marketing strategies in prescription drug use. *Ann World Assn Med Informatics 1981; 1: 13-19*

43. AVORN J, SOUMERAI S: Use of computer-based Medicaid drug data to analyze and correct inappropriate medication use. *J Med Syst*

44. SILVERMAN M, LEE PR: *Pills, Profits and Politics.* University of California Press, 1974

45. MEDEWAR CHARLES: *The Wrong Kind of Medicine?* Consumers' Association and Hodder & Stoughton, 1984

46. CASTLE RN, et al: Antibiotic use at Duke University Medical Center. *JAMA 1977; 237: 2819-2822*

47. PAPADOPOULOS JST: Unpublished data

48. JICK H: The discovery of drug-induced illness. *N Engl J Med 1977; 296: 481-485*

49. BRAITHWAITE J: *Corporate Crime in the Pharmaceutical Industry.* London: Routledge & Kegan Paul, 1984

50. WALLERSTEIN RO, CONDIT PK, KASPER CK, et al: Statewide study of chloramphenicol therapy and fatal aplastic anemia. *JAMA 1969; 208: 2045-2050*

51. HERBST AL, ULFELDER H, POSKANZER DC: Adenocarcinoma of the vagina: association of maternal stilbestrol therapy with tumor appearence in young women. *N Engl J Med 1971; 284: 878-881*

52. SMITH DC, PRENTICE R, THOMSON DJ: Association of exogenous estrogen and endometrial carcinoma. *N Engl J Med 1975; 293: 1164-1167*

53. Boston Collaborative Drug Surveillance Program: Oral contraceptives and venous thromboembolic disease, surgically confirmed gallbladder disease, and breast tumours.

54. GOODMAN and GILLMAN: *The Pharmaceutical Basis of Therapeutics.* 5th ed. 1985

55. NEU HC, HOWREY SP: Testing the physician's knowledge of antibiotic use. *N Engl J Med 1975; 293: 1291-1295*

56. STOLLEY PD, BECKER MH, McEVELLA JD, et al: Drug prescribing and use in an American community. *Ann Int Med 1972; 76: 537-540*

57. ROBERTS AW, VISCONTI JA: The rational and irrational use of systemic antimicrobial drugs. *Amer J Hosp Pharm 1972; 29: 828-834*

58. GROSSINGER R: *Planet Medicine.* Berkeley: North Atlantic Books, 1990: 242

59. GAMBELL and HARRISON: *Urology, Vol 1.* 538-549

60. Editorial: Chronic prostatitis. *Brit Med J 1972; July 1: 1-2*

61. SMITH DR: *General Urology.* 170-173

62. ARYA OP, MALLINSON H, GODDARD AD: Epidemiological and clinical correlates of chlamydial infection of the cervix. *Brit J Vener Dis 1981; 57: 118-124*

63. GUNBY P: Chlamydial infections probably most prevalent of STDs. *Arch Int Med 1983; 143: 1665*

64. MEARES E: Etiology of prostatitis. *Urology (supplement) 1984; 24 : 4-5*

65. THIN RN, SIMMONS PD: Review of results of four regimens for treatment of chronic non-bacterial prostatitis. *Brit J Urology 1983; 55: 519-521*

66. STAMEY TA: Prostatitis. *J Royal Soc Med 1981; 74: 22-33*

67. SCHAEFFER AJ: Pharmacokinetics of antibiotics used in treatment of prostatitis. *Urology (supplement) 1984; 24: 8-9*

68. GOLDFARB M: Clinical efficacy of antibiotics in treatment of prostatitis. *Urology (supplement) 1984; 24: 12-13*

Chapter 1

THE NECESSITY OF A MODEL

> "The myths of Hygieia and Asclepius symbolize the never-ending oscillation between two different points of view in medicine. For the worshippers of Hygieia, health is the natural order of things, a positive attribute to which men are entitled if they govern their lives wisely. According to them, the most important function of medicine is to discover and teach the natural laws which will ensure a healthy mind in a healthy body. More skeptical, or wiser in the ways of the world, the followers of Asclepius believe that the chief role of the physician is to treat disease, to restore health by correcting any imperfections caused by the accidents of birth or life."
>
> Rene Dubos[1]

As far as I know, no serious attempt has been made by anybody in the medical field to present in a comprehensive way a theoretical model of the human body and the way it functions in health and disease. Perhaps the reason is that the human being is so infinitely subtle and complex in its structure and mode of functioning that any attempt to provide a complete model would not only be frustrating but almost impossible. A host of uncertainties looms before us when we consider the fact that the whole organism is much more than a mere composite of its cells, tissues and organs. The seemingly countless and indefinable variables in such a system would seem to frustrate our best efforts to achieve total understanding. Yet established medicine has pretended, or at least has given the impression to the outside world, that it has always acted under the premise of knowing everything about the human organism.

It is for this reason that Henry Simmons ironically states, "We physicians were the experts. The public had little to do or little need to participate in setting medical priorities or making medical decisions; we would look out for their interests; we knew what was best for them." [2]

Medicine, as practiced today, is based more on faith than knowledge, as Mendelsohn aptly states in his book *Confessions of a Medical Heretic:* "You can easily test modern medical religion...by simply asking your doctor 'why?'....Just ask why enough times and sooner or later you'll reach the Chasm of Faith. Your doctor will retreat into the conditioned response that you have no way of... understanding all the wonders he has at his command. Just trust 'him'!" [3]

Other authors who were sensitive enough to perceive the actual situation made similar remarks....

> — "...the patient is... seen as a passive recipient of the intervention, preferably without interference or resistance, since the doctor knows best. (Blum, 1960; Hayes-Bautista and Harveston, 1977) [4]

> — "A patient is seen as a disabled mechanism, and the job of the clinic or hospital is to 'classify, confine and immobilize' the patient." [5]

In reality, what established medicine was offering as a "rationale" for its questionable practices were certain gross models obviously conceived *a posteriori* in order to justify the empirical practices applied in everyday therapeutics. These models were represented as the acme of scientific knowledge.

Following is a short summary of the models which medicine has so far employed.

Since the eighteenth century a mechanistic way of thinking has prevailed in the scientific method which has led to a mechanical approach to the whole problem of health and disease. The body, separated from the rest of the organism, was considered a machine, and as a consequence of such a concept, any imbalance in the machine was considered the effect of a singular causative agent; e.g. a single type of bacterium causing an infectious disease. This theory was called the Koch model. [6]

When this model appeared to be rather superficial, medical scientists formulated a new theory that tended to explain disease as the result of a defect in cellular and molecular functioning. This defect was believed to be caused by an external agent or by a fault in the intrinsic machinery of the cell or in the structure of the molecule. This theory was known as the functional model and was attributed to Virchow. [6,7]

Later, a "diagnostic model" of disease was developed. This model maintained that disease was a totality of symptoms, and if the etiology and pathogenesis were more or less known, the treatment would be rational and specific. This approach contrasted with later knowledge that recognized multiple subforms of every specific disease.[6]

Another model that emerged was the "curative" one, based mainly on the treatment of infectious diseases and vitamin deficiencies.[6]

More recently two more models have been proposed by the contemporary thinkers Weiner and Engel. That conceived by Weiner is more complex than its predecessors; social, cultural and behavioral factors are taken into consideration. The other model by G. L. Engel is even more comprehensive. In his treatise *The Need for a New Medical Model: a Challenge for Biomedicine*, he argues for a new model of medicine, asserting that this is necessary "to provide a basis for understanding the determinants of disease and arriving at rational treatments and patterns of health care; a medical model must also take into account the patient, the social context in which he lives, and the complementary system devised by society." [8]

All these models appear to be rather simplistic, impractical and inadequate in their conception and scope, especially when health and disease are viewed from a broader perspective. Almost all of them seem to have been born out of efforts to justify "fashionable" medical practices rather than to postulate *a priori* a theoretical rationale on which medical thinking and practices could be based. Besides this, the problem of defining health and disease has not been solved, and this is perhaps due to the mechanical and oversimplified concept behind these approaches. Therefore, the necessity for a new theoretical *Model* that expounds upon the complexity and intricate nature of man appears to be crucial today.

REFERENCES:

1. DUBOS R: *Mirage of Health*. New York: Harper & Row, 1971
2. SIMMONS H: An Overview of Public Policy and Infectious Diseases. *Ann Int Med 1978; 89 (part 2): 821-825*
3. MENDELSOHN RS: *Confessions of a Medical Heretic*. Warner Books, 1979; 17

4. PELLETIER K: *Holistic Medicine: From Stress to Optimum Health.* Delta/Seymour Lawrence ed., 1981
5. CARLSON RJ: *The End of Medicine.* New York: Wiley, 1975
6. WEINER H: The illusion of simplicity: The Medical Model Revisited. *Amer J Psychiatry, July 1978; Supplement: 135*
7. VIRCHOW R: *Cellular Pathology.* Translated by Frank Chance. Ann Arbor, MI: Edwards Brothers, 1940
8. ENGEL GL: The need for a new medical model: A challenge for biomedicine. *Science, April 8, 1977; 196(4286): 129-136*

Chapter 2

THE EXISTING SITUATION IN MEDICINE

Medical activities are divided into three separate branches that apparently have no real communication or feedback among themselves.

These three separate branches are:

1. Everyday medicine applied in the hospital and in general practice.
2. Educational centers, universities and post-graduate studies.
3. Research centers.

Of all the three branches the research centers appear to comprise the core of allopathic medicine. The public's expectations of these centers are considerable. The pressures of modern life place a premium on rapid cure and the speedy elimination of symptoms.

In contrast, the educational centers seem to be paralyzed. They have failed to introduce any significant innovations of their own in medical thought, and they have likewise refused to incorporate any of the novel concepts proposed by the alternative health care movement, derogating the alternative ideas as too theoretical or abstract for practical application.

Similarly, medical practitioners have fallen victim to inertia. Despite the discouraging number of therapeutic dead ends encountered in clinical medicine, they have seldom voiced their dissatisfaction with the ineffectiveness of many of the drugs introduced by research centers. By failing to express their complaints, in refraining from upsetting the established sociomedical order, a crucial feedback mechanism among the three branches that could have prevented the current situation has failed to evolve, and the supremacy of medical research has thus been assured.

Research institutions have become the leading medical authorities, and their findings are considered absolute and final. The belief of the system in their "discoveries" has been so great that on certain occasions, when physicians have refused to follow the prescribed regimen, they have been placed in jeopardy of losing their license. Does any medical doctor dare not prescribe chemotherapy for cancer patients today? Yet it is certain that after a period of time such treatment will be outmoded and probably forbidden. Nobody has ever complained about such inconsistencies, even though they cause humanity so much pain and anguish.

Established medicine is pouring millions of dollars, tons of adoration, and very little criticism into these centers. Those few enlightened individuals who raise their voices in protest to various practices run the risk of being ostracized by the very same conservative, "closed" medical society to which they themselves belong.

Meanwhile, there has been a frantic race taking place in the research centers. The opponents to beat are time and pathological agents. That task is quite difficult since the pathogens are so invasive and elusive that no serious researcher dare make any promises or predictions. What they are actually doing at the centers is randomly, without any guiding principles, testing different drugs which would kill or eliminate the pathogen. The most important discoveries of drugs that have been considered really original were made accidentally, e.g. penicillin, aspirin, etc.

This means that the whole process involved in the development of a therapeutic agent is not based on an inductive process, guided by underlying laws and principles, but almost exclusively on the experience of a single individual who has observed certain phenomena in the laboratory. Whereas every other scientific field bases its research upon established laws and principles and then seeks to verify those principles in an organized way, much medical research proceeds in a random, indeterminate and accidental manner. Thus, medicine is more rightly deemed empirical rather than scientific.

Such criticism may sound prejudiced or unfair; nonetheless, the fact remains that most significant therapeutic medical advances owe their advent to fortuitous research findings. New drugs are released and become the new treatment of choice as a result of the intimations of their suitability unveiled by isolated research studies. These findings do not have to comply with any laws of nature. In fact, by ignoring such laws the individual researcher can easily transgress them without guilt or fear of penalty. The penalty is often exacted much later from the patient who must bear the consequences of the new drug's effects.

In Silverman's book *Pills, Profits and Politics,* we find an enlightening passage from testimony given by Dr. Dale Console, a former research director for a large pharmaceutical company, before a Senate committee. He said that:

> "With many of these products, it is clear while they are on the drawing board that they promise no utility. They promise sales. It is not a question of pursuing them because something may come of it... They are pursued simply because there is profit in it... Since so much depends on novelty, drugs change like women's hemlines, and rapid obsolescence is simply a sign of motion, not progress. With a little luck, proper timing, and a good promotion program, any bag of asafoetida with a unique chemical side-chain can be made to look like a wonder drug. The illusion may not last, but it frequently lasts long enough. By the time the doctor learns what the company knew in the beginning, the company has two new products to take the place of the old one...The pharmaceutical industry is unique in that it can make exploitation appear a noble purpose." [1]

Usually what happened was that the researcher's assumptions about the drug remained valid only until it was found that either the drug was a real disaster or that in the long run its side effects were worse than the disease it was originally supposed to cure.

> "In the United States alone, some 1,500,000 of the 30,000,000 patients hospitalized annually are admitted because of adverse reactions to drugs. In some hospitals, as high as 20% of the patients are admitted because of drug-induced disease, and during the one-year period beginning July 1, 1965, at the Montreal General Hospital 25% of the deaths on the public medical service were the result of adverse drug reactions." [2]

> "At least two out of every five patients receiving drugs from their doctors suffer from side effects," [3,4] and "one in every twelve admissions to hospitals is caused by the side effects of treatment." [5]

I do not deny that all this "frantic" research has provided us with interesting insights into the mode of functioning of the human body, but it has managed to produce neither a thoroughly safe drug nor a drug which can cure without side effects.

The reason established medicine has found itself in such a weak position, if not jeopardy, is the fact that its primary research has never been based upon any recognized natural laws or principles governing health and disease. The need to identify such laws or principles is becoming more and more crucial today. All sciences are based on laws of nature, and no one can afford to ignore them, least of all **modern "scientific" medicine.**

REFERENCES:

1. SILVERMAN M, LEE PR: *Pills, Profits & Politics.* University of California Press, 1974
2. MARTIN EW et al: *Hazards of Medication.* Toronto: J. B. Lippincott Co., 1971
3. MARTY CR: *British Medical Journal, 10 November 1979;* 6199: 1194
4. WEITZ M: *Health Shock: A Guide to Ineffective and Hazardous Medical Treatment.* Rome and London: Butler & Tammer Ltd., 1980
5. OWEN D: *In Sickness and In Health.* London: Quartet, 1976

Chapter 3

PRELIMINARY IDEAS

Before presenting my proposed *Model for Health and Disease*, certain clarifications of some basic ideas promoted in this treatise may be necessary. It is for this reason I state, from the very beginning, that in this *Model* **the states of health and disease are considered to be intricately interrelated, and our old concept of disease as a separate and distinct entity should be completely abandoned.**

This idea has been hinted at by professors Manu Kothari and Lopa Mehta, who write, "Medicine has not been able to define what constitutes the normal, be it blood sugar or blood pressure... the differences between the 'normal' and the 'abnormal' are not that between black and white but that between shades of grey, with no dividing line anywhere." [1]

Toon writes in the *Journal of Medical Ethics* of December 1981, "The use of terms 'disease' and 'diseases' has come under increasing scrutiny in recent years... Medicine is leaving behind the idea of 'specific diseases caused by specific agents', if indeed it was ever held."

As Romano also states, "Health and disease are not static entities but are phases of life...." [2]

From such an understanding, we may be talking about "differential health states" rather than distinct, separate states of health and disease. What is meant here is that in the interim from the state of absolute health to the state of near death, there are numerous modifications or substates of health that at certain points in time result in concrete pathology with definite symptomatology. We have all agreed to label these pathological conditions with a specific name, and thus the nomenclature of medicine has developed. Medical doctors will not accept that an individual is suffering from a specific disease unless they discover specific symptomatology which corresponds to their system of nomenclature.

What has never been taken into consideration is that before a patient arrives at a definite pathological state corresponding to an existing disease label, he goes through unexplained states of discomfort or ill health, consisting of several undefined symptoms for which his doctors are unable to prescribe suitable remedies. They can only prescribe a course of treatment if it has been recorded and described previously in the medical literature as a distinct pathological entity.

In the case of chronic disease the problem is that once a patient arrives at such an advanced pathological state, there is usually no possibility of cure; his suffering may be palliated, but by and large he must learn to live with his disease. In reality the patient was in a state of imbalance for quite a long time before manifesting the gross pathology which we call disease. It is the failure of doctors to incorporate the earlier states of imbalance within their disease framework that has prevented medicine from implementing effective preventive care.

The *Model* also presupposes that there is an "ideal" state of health (in reality unattainable), and also that all individuals find themselves within a "continuum" where at any given time they are in a "relative" condition of health.

The *Model* will not be examining the human being's anatomical structure and physiology. That has already been done quite extensively, although a lot still has to be learned. Rather, it will be examining the dynamic, complex structure and interactions **of interrelated energy fields and organizational patterns**. This *Model* is strongly based on what Einstein has said concerning all matter: "We may therefore regard matter as being constituted by the regions of space in which the field is extremely intense...there is no place in this new kind of physics both for the field and matter, for the field is the only reality." [3]

The *Model* will also take into consideration the **individuality** and **uniqueness** of the human being as well as his individualized response to stimuli. The fingerprint of an individual is uniquely "his" and his alone—it is his mark, his seal of identification. We know that fingerprint patterns are specific genetic combinations that are unique in every case. These same fingerprints that identify an individual as Mr. John Doe on the physical level have their counterparts on the emotional and intellectual levels.

If it were possible that someone could objectively observe humanity, all human beings would look alike. Established medicine has generally treated all human beings alike, as if they were identical machines with an identical defect that needed an identical remedy. This whole concept has been aggressively promoted and promulgated as the ultimate of scientific attainment. The question that should arise in medicine is "can we afford to ignore the principle of individualization in treating diseased individuals?" But Weiner states, "People are infinitely variable; psychological polymorphism is limitless, so one cannot label people accurately. Diagnosis is fruitless, classification difficult." [4]

Even today, the trend in research laboratories is to find a drug to **cure** cancer, AIDS, epilepsy, etc., never to cure the "individual that has cancer, AIDS or epilepsy."

So far it has not been understood that one individual with "cancer" **can** be cured while another with the same type of cancer cannot; an individual with epilepsy can be treated successfully and another cannot; and I even dare say one with AIDS can be cured while another cannot. In medical literature, spontaneous cures for all diseases, even the most severe ones, have been described and millions of cures have taken place outside of established medicine—the result of alternative methods of treatment. [5-21]

One must ask certain key questions in order to explain certain facts about the AIDS virus. Why is it that certain individuals will not even be carriers of the virus in spite of coming in contact with it, while others who are carriers will never develop AIDS? Why will some individuals get the virus and succumb to it within a short period of time, while others succumb to it at a much later date?

A simple example of this concerns the Hepatitis B virus. There are millions of carriers of the Hepatitis B virus. Nevertheless, the majority of these people remain carriers and do not develop any of the variety of diseases associated with it. Others may develop any of the following diseases—acute hepatitis, chronic hepatitis, immunological abnormalities or deficiencies, liver cirrhosis or primary hepatic carcinoma.

Established medicine has never considered the "constitution" of the sick individual a matter of therapeutic concern.

There are a number of cases that demonstrate how drugs, given to sensitive patients without regard for those sensitivities, have held disastrous consequences for the patient. Some of these side effects, selected at random from current medical journals,[22] are:

— posterior subcapsular cataracts in steroid treated children
— blindness from betamethasone eye drops
— poisoning with boric acid
— red cell aplasia resulting from antituberculosis therapy
— intracranial hemorrhage with amphetamines[23]
— liver injury from halothane[24]
— fatal hepatitis due to indomethacin[25,26]
— severe reaction from anticholinesterase eye drops[27]
— hepatotoxicity and fatalities after methoxyflurane anesthesia[28,29]
— hyperglycemia from trioxazine[30]
— lung diseases caused by various drugs, teratogenic effects from various drugs[31,32]
— intestinal ulceration with mefenamic acid[33]
— fatal nephritis with phenacetin[34]
— permanent deafness with ethacrynic acid[35]
— allergic reactions with antimicrobials[36-39]
— visual impairment with an antimalarial[40]
— thrombophlebitis with oral contraceptives[41]
— physical and psychological dependence with methamphetamine[42]
— delayed, severe, prolonged and fatal effects from radiopaque diagnostic drugs.

We find in the medical literature articles by responsible people such as Illich,[43] Burnet,[44] Dubos,[45] Goldblatt,[46] Platt,[47] Carlson,[48] McKeown,[49] Knowles,[50] etc., stressing the importance of the "constitution" as a whole. Unfortunately, since their ideas have always been judged on theoretical grounds, they have never been applied in day-to-day practice.

The concept that the "constitution" as a whole must be supported and strengthened therapeutically has never been pursued in the research laboratories, although the medical establishment has pretended to recognize its importance. What research has pursued are the "invaders" that thrive in this "constitution."

It appears that for the last forty years intelligent scientists have wasted precious effort and millions of dollars in the elusive quest for a "panacea" for the diseases of humanity. One medicine for every disease was not good enough, but one medicine to cure all diseases was the "quixotic" dream of every scientist—a dream originating from a wrong perception of who the diseased individual really was.

"Our problems in infectious diseases get bigger, more expensive, and more hazardous. We are at the point where thoughtful observers are questioning not whether we are in the post-infectious era, but whether, on balance, society is much better off than we were 40 years ago, despite our hundreds of new antibiotics, hundreds of millions of prescriptions, and billions of dollars of expense. In view of all the evidence, a positive answer to this question can no longer be given with confidence; it is a legitimate question....

"It appears that we could double or halve our total health expenditures without significantly affecting the nation's health. It seems that in the United States there is no longer any important relation between the amount of money spent on traditional health care and the results achieved." [51]

In spite of utter failure and frustration coming from within medical ranks, the "quest" is still obstinately pursued, without a change in the way of thinking, without anybody seriously challenging the principles underlying current research methods.

On the contrary, some medical authorities still insist that the assumption is valid that general medicine is beneficial and leads to a decline in mortality rate and an increase in life expectancy. This belief, to say the least, is questionable today, and I am sure it will be invalidated in a few years' time. As Dubos wrote in 1968, "While they have done much in the prevention and treatment of a few specific diseases, they have so far failed to increase true longevity or to create positive health." [52]

Simmons states, "Most of the major improvements in longevity in this century, and the dramatic decrease in mortality from infectious diseases specifically, occurred long before we began our massive spending for health care and antibiotic drugs. McKinlay suggests that only about 3.5% of the fall of the overall death rate in this century can reasonably be attributed to medical measures including medical interventions in the major infectious diseases...It seems that the major impact on these diseases is likelier to come from changes in lifestyle, behavior, and the environment than from traditional medical care." [51]

McKeown, the reknowned medical thinker and researcher, states that the contribution of clinical medicine to the prevention of death and the increase in life expectancy in the past three centuries was smaller than the influence of the solution to problems of malnutrition, of water and food shortages and of the disproportion between rates of reproduction and the basic resources of life.

Another example of drug "futility" is exemplified in the following statement by McKeown, "...the mortality from tuberculosis fell sharply from the time when it was first recorded; since then, a large part of the decline occurred before the introduction of effective treatment in 1947." [49] (*Figure 3*) However, Drews, the director of the research department at SANDOZ, presented a misleading diagram. Only a portion of the general diagram was shown in order to prove that the course of tuberculosis was affected drastically by the introduction of chemotherapy (*Figure 4*).

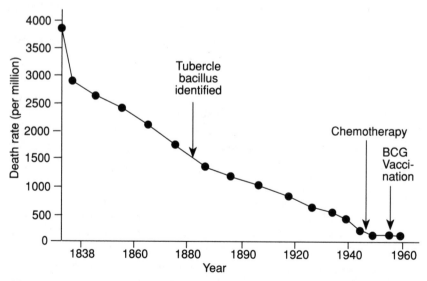

Figure 3: Respiratory tuberculosis: mean annual death rates (standardized to 1901 population): England and Wales.

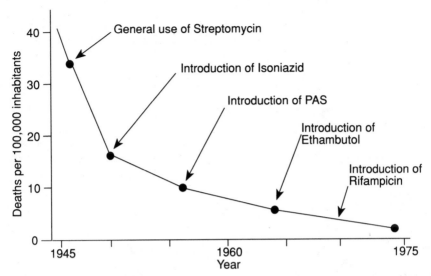

Figure 4: Decrease in the mortality rates from tuberculosis between 1945-49. From: Drews, J: *Historische und Zukuenftige Perspectiven in der Pharmazeutischen Forschung.* Triangel-Sandoz, 22 (1983).

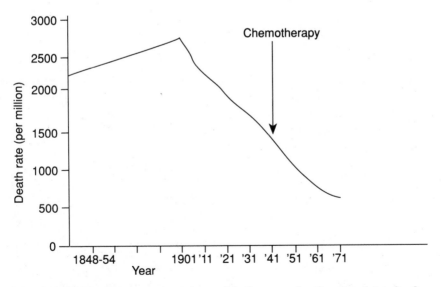

Figure 5: Bronchitis, pneumonia, and influenza: death rates (standardized to 1901 population): England and Wales.

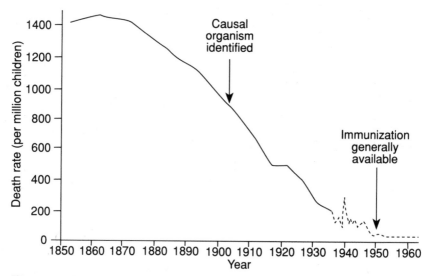

Figure 6: Whooping cough: death rates of children under 15: England and Wales.

The "true" diagram (*Figure 3*) shows the decline of tuberculosis had already begun before chemotherapy was introduced. Drews, in his book, misleads us in giving only part of the diagram.[49]

Clinical trials and clinical experience leave no doubt that antibiotics were not the main cause for the decrease of bacterial pneumonia, as McKeown writes: "What these data show (*Figure 5*) is that the mortality rate from respiratory diseases certified initially under bronchitis, influenza and pneumonia, and later under pneumonia, was decreasing since the beginning of the century and that its continued decline, after 1935, was not due primarily to chemotherapy."

In England and Wales, the death rate from whooping cough has declined since 1860 (*Figure 6*). The effectiveness of treatment is still in doubt, and the more important issue is the contribution of immunization, as mortality had fallen to a low level before immunization was introduced.

With some variation in timing, the history of measles has been rather similar to that of whooping cough (*Figure 7*). The death rate fell continuously from about 1915; treatment of

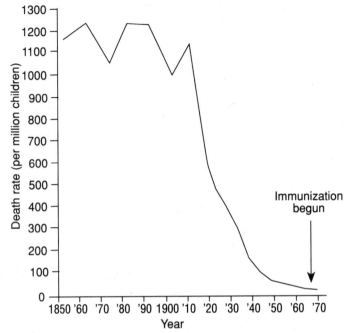

Figure 7: Measles: death rates of children under 15: England and Wales.
Haldane JBS, *Science and Life, 1968; London, Pemberton: 65*

secondary infections has been possible since 1935; and mortality
was at a low level before immunization was introduced.

From these examples, and many more cited in the various
texts and journals, it is clear that we have been wrongly
attributing the above-cited improvements in society's health to
allopathic pharmaceuticals.

It is my assumption that if we do not change our orientation
now we may not be able to secure our own survival on this planet.

REFERENCES:

1. KOTHARI ML, METHA LA: The trans-science aspects of disease and
    death. *Perspect Biol Med 1981; 24: 658-666*
2. ROMANO J: Basic Orientation and Education of the Medical Student.
    JAMA 1950; 143: 490-412
3. CAPRA F: *The Tao of Physics.* New York: Bantam, 1977

4. WEINER H: The illusion of simplicity: The Medical Model revisited. *Am J Psychiatry, July 1978; 135: Supplement 27-33*

5. ABESHOUSE BS, SCHERLIS I: Spontaneous disappearence of retrogression of bladder neoplasms: Review of the literature and report of three cases. *Urol Cutan Rev 1951; 55(1)*

6. ALLEN EP: Malignant melanoma, spontaneous regression after pregnancy. *Brit Med J 1955; 2: 1955*

7. ALVAREZ WC: The spontaneous regression of cancer. *Geriatrics 1967; 22: 88-90*

8. BAKER HW: Spontaneous regression of malignant melanoma. *Amer Surg 1964; 30: 825-831*

9. BARTLEY O, HULTQUIST GT: Spontaneous regression of hypernephromas. *Acta Path Microb 1950; 80: 197*

10. BESWICK IP, QVIST G: Spontaneous regression of cancer. *Brit Med J 1963; 2: 1842*

11. BIERMAN EO: Spontaneous regression of malignant disease. *JAMA 1959; 170: 1842*

12. BONIUC M, GIRALD LJ: Spontaneous regression of bilateral retinoblastoma. *Trans Amer Acad Opthal Otolaryng 1969; 73: 194-198*

13. BOYD W: *The Spontaneous Regression of Cancer.* Springfield, IL: Charles C Thomas, 1966

14. DAO TL: Regression of pulmonary metastases of a breast cancer. *AMA Arch Surg 1962; 84: 574*

15. EVERSON TC: Spontaneous regression of cancer. *Progr Clin Cancer 1967; 3: 79-85*

16. LEGIER JF: Spontaneous regression of primary bile duct carcinoma. *Cancer 1964; 17: 730*

17. LESHAN L: *How to Meditate.* New York: Bantam, 1974 (a)

18. LESHAN L: *The Medium, the Mystic, and the Physicist.* New York: Viking, 1974 (b)

19. NELSON DH: Spontaneous regression of cancer. *Clinic Radiology 1962; 13: 138*

20. SELIGMAN AM: A review of Everson, Tilden, Cole,Waner: Spontaneous regression of cancer: A study and abstracts of reports in the world medical literature and of personal communications concerning spontaneous regression of malignant disease. *JAMA 1966; 198(6), 680*

21. SIMMONTON OC, MATHEWS-SIMMONTON S, CREIGHTON J: *Getting Well Again.* Los Angeles: J. P. Tarcher, 1978

22. MARTIN EW et al: *Hazards of Medication.* Toronto: JB Lippincott Co., 1971

23. GOODMAN SB, BECKER DP: Intracranial hemorrhage associated with amphetamine abuse. *JAMA 1970; 122: 480*

24. Halothane and liver injury. *Med Let 1968; 10: 7-8*

25. GUERRA M: Toxicity of indomethacin. *JAMA 1967; 200: 552*

26. KELSEY WM, SCARY JM: Fatal hepatitis probably due to indomethacin. *JAMA 1967; 199: 586-587*

27. KINYON GE: Anticholinesterase eye drops—need for caution. *New Engl J Med 1969; 280: 53*

28. KLEIN NC, JEFFRIES GH: Hepatotoxicity after methoxyflurane administration. *JAMA 1966; 197: 1037-1039*

29. PANNER BJ, FREEMAN RB, ROTH-MOYO LA: Toxicity following methoxyflurane anesthesia: Clinical and pathological observations in two fatal cases. *JAMA 1970; 214: 86-90*

30. KRUMHOLZ WV, CHIPPS HI, MERLIS S: Clinical effects of trioxazine with a case report of hyperglycemia as a side effect. *J Clin Pharmacol 1967; 7: 108-110*

31. McCUTCHEON S: Teratogenic drugs. *Pharma Index 1969; 11: 5-8*

32. MEADOW SR: Anticonvulsant drugs and congenital abnormalities. *Lancet 1968; 2: 1296*

33. Trends in centrally acting drugs. *Pharma Index 1969; 12: 5-12 (May), 4-8 (June), 4-7 (July)*

34. MOOLTEN SE, SMITH LB: Fatal nephritis in chronic phenacetin poisoning. *Amer J Med 1960; 28: 127-134*

35. PILLAY VKG, SCHWARTZ FD, AIMI K: Transient and permanent deafness following treatment with ethacrynic acid in renal failure. *Lancet 1969; 1: 77-79*

36. Principal toxic, allergic, and other adverse effects of antimicrobial drugs. *Med Let 1968; 10: 73-76*

37. SANDERS DY: Rash associated with ampicillin in infectious mononucleosis. *Clin Pediatr 1969; 8: 47-48*

38. SMITH LW, JOHNSON JE, III, CLUFF LE: Studies on the epidemiology of adverse drug reactions: II. An evaluation of penicillin allergy. *N Engl J Med 1966; 274: 998-1002*

39. STEWART GT: Allergenic residues in penicillins. *Lancet 1967; 1: 1177-1183*

40. ROTHERMICH DY: Visual impairment from antimalarial drug. *N Engl J Med 1966; 275: 1383*

41. SLUGGET J, LAWSON JP: Side effects of oral contraceptives. *Lancet 1965; 2: 612*

42. SMITH DE: Physical versus psychological dependence and tolerance in high-dose methamphetamine abuse. *Clin Toxic 1969; 2: 99-103*

43. ILLICH I: *Medical Nemesis: The Expropriation of Health.* London: Boyars, 1975

44. BURNET FM: *Genes, Dreams and Realities.* Aylesbury: MTP, 1971

45. DUBOS RJ: *The Dreams of Reason: Science and Utopias.* New York: Columbia Univ. Press, 1961

46. GOLDBLATT DP: Modern medicine's shortcomings: can we really conquer disease? *Perspect Biol Med 1977; 20: 450-456*

47. PLATT R: *Private and Controversial.* London: Boyars, 1975

48. CARLSON RJ: *The End of Medicine.* New York: Wiley, 1978

49. McKEOWN T: *The Role of Medicine: Dream, Mirage or Nemesis?* Basil Blackwell Publisher Ltd., 1979

50. KNOWLES JH: *Doing Better and Feeling Worse.* New York: Norton, 1977

51. SIMMONS H: An overview of public policy and infectious diseases. *Ann Inter Med 1978; (Part 2): 821-825*

52. DUBOS RJ: *So Human an Animal.* Charles Scribner's Sons, 1968

53. DREWS J: *Historische und Zukuenftige Perspectiven in der Pharmazeutischen Forschung.* Triangel-Sandoz, 22 (1983) s. 189

Chapter 4

THE ENERGY COMPLEX OF THE HUMAN BODY

1. The human body is an energy complex that generates all forms of familiar energies—electric, magnetic, thermal, kinetic and electromagnetic —which can easily be detected by simple devices of which the most sophisticated is the electroencephalograph. But there are also other types of subtle energies that have not yet been defined and which relate primarily to the mental, emotional and instinctual levels of the human being.

Today, nobody can deny the existence of **mental, emotional** and **sexual energies**.[1-16] We all understand and perceive when a certain person has a strong mental energy (M_e), that his thought patterns are strong, well organized, coherent, easily communicated, and therefore effective in influencing others.

On the other hand we may note a person's mental weakness, the chaotic way he expresses his ideas, the lack of organizational patterns in his thinking processes, and how much less effective he is in communicating his thoughts.

We frequently hear of extrasensory experiences or experience them ourselves. We can "tune in" to another person's thought pattern before he has verbally communicated this thought to us. In the Far East, especially in India, mind reading is a common phenomenon among those who have prepared themselves for such a task. Krishna Menon, India's Minister of External Affairs, was renowned for his capacity to read the minds of those who visited him for a request.

Mental power seems to be a perceptible energy with a specific vibrational frequency that can be transmitted by energy particles under specialized conditions and thus be "received" by other similar "mental apparati." The fact that this kind of energy is not defined in the academic texts does not make it non-existent.

Most of us live with a constant flow of thoughts occurring in our mind. The greatest part of our waking hours, and thus our very existence, revolves around the constant generation of these thought patterns. We cannot afford to ignore such an important aspect of ourselves, especially when this area can be affected by the application of a therapeutic system. Yet established medicine has completely bypassed this important aspect in its search for a "cure" and has pretended that it did not exist. When it tested the new drugs, it very seldom investigated how deeply and in what manner they affected the human mind.

"The psychiatrists reminded their fellow scientists that the body's own self-regulatory functions may be taken over by the drugs used...

"Even hormones primarily affect the brain; the Pill, in large therapeutic doses, caused temporary psychosis in 4 percent of the wives of armed forces personnel being treated for infertility. Drugs with specific ambitions— diuretics, antihistamines—may be indirectly psychoactive...

"They began pushing amphetamines as energy aids, and by the mid-1950s there were half a million amphetamine addicts in Japan. Fifty thousand cases of amphetamine psychosis had been reported." [17]

"The worst offenders in producing depression are members of the reserpine type of alkaloids... Hypertensive patients receiving these alkaloids are most likely to become highly depressed even to the point of suicide...

"The anticholinergics such as benztropine, biperidine and procyclidine have a potential to produce delirium...

"Agitation, auditory, gustatory, tactile and visual hallucinations and sometimes disorientation have occurred with procaine penicillin...

"Psychosis or neurosis have been caused by a variety of drugs...

"Manifestations commonly observed are delusions, paranoid behavior and various kinds of hallucinations. These closely resemble the symptoms of schizophrenia." [18]

Certain antibiotics substantially increased senile brain disease and Down's syndrome through treatment of previously fatal complications such as infection. "Gruenberg presents data that indicate a doubling in prevalence of these conditions in recent decades. He terms this phenomenon the failures of success." [19]

It is true that this field of research is difficult and hard to investigate properly, but this is not a good enough reason for dismissing the damage caused by these drugs on the mental and emotional planes. The emotional and mental changes brought about cannot always be detected anatomically or by a microscope, but they have been related by patients experiencing these changes; many times their experiences were dismissed or ignored by researchers.

It is even easier to perceive the existence and power of **emotional energy** because it is on a grosser level than mental energy. Everybody has had the experience of being in the presence of a very angry person and perceiving the discharge of aggressive energy flowing from that person. This is even more evident when two people are extremely angry at one another. There may be complete silence, words may not be spoken, but there are negative, aggressive vibrations in the air felt by many of those present. Enormous flow of a specific, emotional energy (E_e) is generated in such a situation that nobody can ignore or dismiss.

Another situation in which a lot of emotional energy is generated is when two people fall in love. This energy is specific, directed toward the loved one, and can be perceived without words; there is a total communication of love to the other person.

Everybody will say that someone who is upset is in a state of emotional agitation. Yet established medicine has never researched the type of mental or emotional upsets produced by the different pharmaceutical products. Later we shall try to show that these mental and emotional areas suffer the most damage from chemical drugs.

The reason why established medicine does not consider these elements lies in the very structure and process of the experiment itself. Scientists have to ignore individualized reactions to the drug under examination; otherwise, they would not be able to repeat an experiment. Even today it is apparent that medical research operates and bases its research on a "mechanical" concept of the human being. [20,21]

The **sexual energy's** potential is very obvious in everyday life, so much so that I feel I do not have explain it in any great depth. It remains on an even grosser or more material level than emotional energy. Examples of sexual energy are commonplace. We are all familiar with cases where someone is very tired and has no energy. He meets a woman that he loves and energy is produced in this encounter. Not only does he now have energy but he feels rejuvenated.

For years advertisers have acknowledged and very successfully utilized sexuality and the energy it produces in their marketing campaigns. Such is the great power of sexual energy.

2. The human being is constructed of three basic planes of energy fields or organizational patterns:
   a. The mental–spiritual plane
   b. The emotional–psychic plane
   c. The physical–material plane that includes instincts and the five senses

In treating the whole person, a medical system has to precisely define all these planes as well as the way they interrelate.

In this way we see how important one level is in comparison with another, how important a function or organ is within a plane. This leads us even further in determining the hierarchical importance of different functions, organs and systems within a plane.

As we shall see later, this *Model* suggests that disease be more precisely called "imbalance of the organism." This generic term implies that an undefined disturbance can shift from one plane to another, from one system to another, and from one organ to another. The degree of health of an individual will eventually be determined by an evaluation of the disturbance on all these levels.

During the process of treatment, if we observe that the disturbance is moving from more important planes to less important ones and from more important and central organs to less important and peripheral ones, then we know that a real cure is taking place. If the opposite direction is observed, if the disturbance is going towards deeper levels, then we have to acknowledge that a suppression is taking place rather than a cure. We shall talk about this idea again during the exposition of the *Model* of health and disease. Now we will define the importance of each plane.

The Mental–Spiritual Plane

In the exposition that follows I do not claim to cover this subject exhaustively, but only to give information sufficient to make my point concerning the structure of this *Model*. Exploring the mental–spiritual aspect of man, defining it and trying to understand its structure and the subtlety of its operation, requires a book by itself. Here I shall only present the rudimentary facts concerning these levels in health and disease.

I have included the human being's spiritual side in the mental level because I consider it to be the highest part of this plane. This aspect, though, is not fully developed in all people. It is an aspect that permits evolution or improvement and exists at the least in a "dormant state" in all individuals. For instance, for primitive people it is the primordial fear of the supernatural or unknown that leads them to the most rudimentary elements of religion and to the formation of a spiritual nature.

According to some sociologists and psychologists the "fear of death" has become a substantial factor in our "civilized" western society. This is also clearly depicted in established medicine's attitude and edicts concerning death. Medicine's whole philosophy in trying to cure people and prevent death at whatever cost to the individual, his family and society has a lot to do with this fear of death.

The more evolved the individual, the more developed is his spiritual aspect. Once the spiritual plane is awakened, the individual is driven by an inner desire, an inner quest to find answers to certain essential issues. The basic questions we usually ask are:

— "Who am I?"
— "Where am I going?"
— "What is the purpose of my life?"
— "What is my mission in this world?"
— "What is God?"
— "What is Truth?" etc.

At times the answers to these questions come to a blessed few of us in the form of sublime mystical experiences.

The positive expression of this plane is the development of the individual's spiritual consciousness; its negative expression is the deterioration of consciousness and consequent degeneration into moral and ethical chaos.

When this spirituality develops in a natural and healthy way, one feels a deep sense of humility and is inspired to selfless service. In addition, a spiritually developed individual enjoys a profound sense of mental quietude. But when spirituality is developed in an unhealthy way, negative qualities such as arrogance, selfishness, uneasiness and a disturbing sense of guilt appear.

If medicinal drugs destroy this plane of existence, it is assumed that this definitely constitutes a suppression rather than a cure, even if the physical pathology has been temporarily relieved. Here is an example: A man seeks treatment for his rheumatoid arthritis, and after a year or two of treatment, he finds that his joint pains are better but that he has lost all sense of happiness and freedom; his ability to reflect on the essential issues of life has been minimized or lost. According to the *Model* of health and disease, this treatment would be called **suppressive**. It is suppressive because, while the physical ailments are getting better, the man is being destroyed on a deeper level.

Other aspects of the mental plane further down the hierarchical scale than the spiritual are the thinking processes—the abilities to compare, calculate, synthesize, analyze, communicate, perceive, create and express ideas, do abstract thinking, etc. In essence, one can say that the **mental plane is the part of the organism that registers changes in perception and understanding**. A disturbance of these functions constitutes mental symptoms or mental derangement. In order for the mental faculties to be considered healthy they should possess the following qualities:

1. **Clarity**
2. **Coherence**
3. **Creativity**

I will assume that clarity and coherence are self-explanatory and will proceed to the definition of creativity. By **healthy creativity** I mean any kind of creative act, regardless of artistic merit—the building of a factory, the production of a piece of furniture, setting up a shop, making a piece of art, repairing a television set, etc. But for such activities to be considered healthy, they must be motivated by two essential intentions:

1. Serving oneself by satisfying one's own needs, ultimately to promote self-evolution.
2. Serving others at the same time with the same objectives.

It is important that the individual feels happiness in serving others to the same degree that he feels happiness in serving himself. An individual who is healthy always considers the consequences that his actions have upon others.

Our educational system elevates the merits of logic and scientific excellence at the expense of morality and ethics. Few curricula contain classes in morality and ethics, subjects that should rightfully dominate our thought. As a consequence, our educational system has unwittingly endorsed deception. For example, many brilliant legal minds seek to gain advantage by devious and clever manipulation of the laws, unconscious of the ethical implications of their behavior. Such instances are far from sporadic; they are, in fact, endemic in our society. Rather than glorifying that which is just and morally upright, our society often seems to discourage and scorn the adherence to moral imperatives. Is it possible to promote health in such an environment?

We must remember that the mind **feeds and grows on ideas,** and if the ideas that are accepted and nurtured by the mind are false or destructive, the individual is actually "taking in poisonous food" that is eventually going to undermine the spiritual plane of his existence. It is somewhat analogous to somebody eating "junk food" all the time; the end result will be the destruction of his physical body. Are not such diseases as AIDS and cancer to be expected in such a society?

A disturbing phenomenon of contemporary society is the aggressive pursuit of excessive wealth through exploitation of others. This acquired wealth is then frequently squandered on lavish self-indulgence. Philanthropic concerns evaporate in the heat of such greed. Individuals caught up in this modern phenomenon may possess mental clarity and coherence; their capabilities in the business world attest to that. However, on the deepest levels of the mental–spiritual plane such persons are very sick; all of their "creative" actions are selfishly motivated, serving only themselves.

Unfortunately, such widespread greed and selfishness is a sign of the spiritual crisis of our times and is primarily responsible for the increasing "insanity" in our western societies. The insecurity, tremendous anxiety, anger, hurriedness, superficiality, insensitiveness, callousness, competitiveness, aggressiveness, irritability, paranoia, criminality, etc., are all results of the deep mental and spiritual imbalance which is so prevalent in our times. We must learn where the responsibility for this imbalance lies.

The question we have to ask is: How many of these mental aberrations are due to the chemical drugs that we have ingested in many forms over the last thirty to forty years? The answer may not only be surprising, but appalling.

The Emotional–Psychic Plane

Defining and expounding on the emotional–psychic plane is not an easy task, and the same remarks apply here as for the mental plane. Here only the rudiments of these planes will be described and only in conjunction with health and disease.

Simply put, one can say that the **emotional plane is that part which generates and registers emotions.**

We all experience a wide range of emotional states in different degrees, those emotions ranging between such polar opposites as love/hatred, joy/sadness, calmness/anxiety, trust/distrust, courage/fear, security/insecurity, etc. What we usually experience are all the degrees of intermediate emotional states between these polar opposites.

To the degree that an individual nurtures positive feelings, we can say that he is healthy on the emotional level.

Positive feelings will tend to bring about a sense of happiness. Yet as has been said before, consistently positive emotions are an impossibility. Opposing states, between which we all vacillate, are part of the very nature of the emotional realm.

The more negative feelings an individual experiences, the less healthy he is on the emotional level; and the extent of his emotional ill health will be proportionately reflected in a pervading sense of unhappiness. If one wants to find out how sick he is on this plane, he must make note of his negative feelings such as apathy, anger, anxiety, hatred, envy, depression, disappointment, dissatisfaction, etc. The size of his inventory of such feelings will reveal the degree of unhealthiness, negativity and unhappiness in which he is living. It is an amazing law of nature that negative feelings are more or less necessary to impel the individual to overcome weaknesses and faults on this plane.

A characteristic quality of positive feelings ranging from simple affection to sublime ecstasy is that they give the individual a sense of oneness, a feeling of unification with the Universe and with others. This is because it is in the nature of love to bring people closer together, to unite, to overcome feelings of separateness.

Negative feelings tend to generate a sense of separation, a feeling of isolation of the individual from the world in general and from other people in particular, as hatred separates and destroys unions.

In the emotional plane we can also include the psychic part of the human being, which is expressed through the subconscious and the intuitive element. This part of the human being is very powerful, and its impressions have a lot to do with the manifestation of disease.

In diseased individuals the subconscious is usually loaded with powerful negative impressions that can hold and manipulate the individual's behavior for quite a long time. Healthy people immediately deal with everyday challenges and impressions and do not let negative feelings settle in their subconscious. Therefore, healthy people usually have a "light" or "clean" subconscious that gives them a greater degree of freedom.

It is doubtful whether even today the significance of the emotional level in triggering disease is fully understood. It is my assumption that in the western world this part of the individual is the weakest; furthermore, it is the most neglected part in our cultural and educational system.

Education, with its emphasis on the mental level, has focused inordinately on developing certain areas of the mind to the exclusion of others. Our educational system has ignored our emotional level, leaving everybody to improvise. Even worse, our societal structures seem to promote the idea that emotions do not exist, or at best, should not be displayed. In certain families the parents unwittingly teach the children to stifle their emotions. "Stop crying" is a command that almost every American child has heard at one point or another. It has never been realized that crying might have spared this child a lot of health problems later on in life.

Emotions **feed on impressions.**

If the food is poisonous, if the impressions that an individual receives are horrid, frightful or even malignant—as when a child witnesses his parents viciously fighting, or watches violence and injustice on television and in real life, or witnesses the aggression and lack of harmony in large cities, for example—then the emotional body will be quickly and deeply disturbed. Can we grow up with a strong, healthy emotional plane under such circumstances? The answer for most of us is no, we cannot.

This is the reason why the weakest, most vulnerable aspect of the people of western civilization is their emotional level.

A comparison of death rates attributed to suicide (per 100,000 of the standard population) can give us an impression of the comparative imbalance between developed and developing countries on the emotional-psychic level. [20,21,22]

Nobody has so far remarked on the significant discrepancy between the high incidence of suicide (emotional disturbances) in the developed and Communist bloc countries (in spite of nationwide health coverage) and the low incidence in developing countries that have poor health coverage from the perspective of "established" medicine.

It is apparent that countries with widespread health coverage, be it voluntary or enforced, have inflicted terrible emotional disturbances on their people, the climax of which is depicted in the rates of suicide.

Western countries (developed):

	1979	1980	1981	1982	1983	1984	1985
Denmark	—	—	—	29.1	28.2	—	—
Austria	—	—	—	26.8	26.0	26.2	—
Switzerland	—	—	—	—	—	23.4	23.7
FDR	—	—	—	19.9	—	18.7	—
France	—	—	19.2	—	—	—	21.3
Sweden	—	—	—	18.7	—	18.8	—
Canada	14.7	—	—	14.7	—	—	—
USA	—	12.0	—	12.3	—	—	—

Eastern European countries:

	1979	1980	1981	1982	1983	1984	1985
Hungary	—	—	—	42.7	—	45.0	—
Czechoslovakia	—	—	20.7	—	19.9	—	—
Yugoslavia	—	—	17.4	17.4	—	—	—
Bulgaria	—	—	—	15.2	13.1	16.6	—

The USSR, Rumania and the Democratic Republic of Germany have not given any rates.

Developing countries:

	1979	1980	1981	1982	1983	1984	1985
Malta	—	—	—	0.4	—	—	0.4
Kuwait	—	—	—	0.1	—	—	1.1
The Bahamas	—	—	1.1	—	—	—	—
Barbados	—	—	—	—	—	1.6	—
Mauritius	—	—	1.9	2.0	—	—	—
Mexico	—	—	—	2.2	—	—	—
Panama	—	—	—	—	2.5	1.8	—
Greece	—	—	—	3.5	—	3.3	—
Dominican Republic	—	—	4.0	—	—	—	—
Spain	—	—	—	—	—	4.7	—
Costa Rica	—	6.8	—	—	—	—	—

As we may assume from the above statistics, developed countries whose populations have consumed tremendous amounts of allopathic drugs have high suicide rates, while underdeveloped countries have significantly lower rates. According to my hypothesis, the emotional plane, which is the weakest and the least-trained of the three planes, has been affected more easily and more severely by the consumption of such enormous quantities of drugs, something that did not occur in underdeveloped countries because they could not afford all these medicines.

These statistics point out the possibility that diseases, or rather "imbalances", will easily move on to the emotional plane under the stress of chemical drugs and cause a host of very painful psychological conditions, such as anxiety or phobic neuroses, depression, manic-depression, and in short, all those emotional disturbances that are so prevalent in our modern western societies today.

The Physical Plane

The physical body is the part of the human being that has received the most attention. It has been analyzed, dissected, examined in its anatomical structure and physiology to an unprecedented degree. It is the most tangible part and therefore the most readily available for investigation. Yet I do not believe that it has given up all its secrets. In fact, it is very doubtful whether its inherent laws have been understood at all.

It is a matter of great curiosity how it was possible for medical science to continue interfering deeply with the mechanisms of the physical body without previously seeking to understand the laws and principles on which its physiology and functioning are based. In their investigations and interference with the physical body of man, scientists have only seen a small part of the whole; many things have escaped their scrutiny, and all the "hints" that were forthcoming were totally ignored. Nobody seemed to take into consideration how the organism reacted as a whole; they seemed interested only in immediate, short-term effects while focusing upon isolated phenomena—solitary links in an infinite chain of biological processes.

As a consequence of such a blind attitude, we have witnessed the well-known side effects of massive medication; and I believe we shall eventually recognize that these side effects are much worse, deeper, more enduring, and in general more devastating than was originally thought.

Dr. Martin aptly expresses this idea when he says, "Long-term therapy, or sometimes short-term therapy, with a toxic medication used to treat a specific disease may cause another disease. The given disease-producing medication may affect a healthy organ, but is more likely to injure a diseased organ or throw a subclinical or controlled state into a full-blown case." [18]

Strangely enough, even though allopathic medicine is not based on any natural principles or laws and despite its lack of etiological validity, it has been widely accepted without substantial objection. This is due in part to the fact that it fits the needs and demands of western societies.

This new *Model* will attempt to provide some basic thoughts concerning the overall function of the human being and stipulate some of its laws, and principles; but, as I said before, it will be far from a final answer to such complicated issues.

The truth of the matter, as we have already seen, is that the physical body is not the whole reality of our existence, and any medical system that does not take other important levels of the organism into consideration is doomed to failure.

Established, "scientific" medicine can learn a lot from alternative medicine, but it has never turned to those disciplines for help or "hints." On the contrary, established medicine has made desperate attempts to squelch any serious efforts on the part of alternative medicine to advance its ideas.

Nobody denies the attainments of established medical research, but what is implied here is that in haste to afford relief, medical science has ignored certain aspects that are absolutely vital in understanding the human body in its entirety. The long-term results of this practice have proven disastrous.

In despair, people turned to alternatives, and so the Holistic movement appeared. Medical science will now reluctantly, perhaps even under coercion, learn from it.

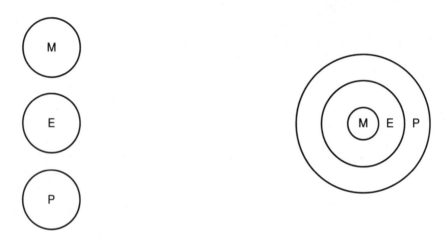

Figure 8: The three planes of being: Mental, Emotional and Physical.

3. A hierarchical relationship exists among the three planes

It appears that the organism, by some intricate mechanism, maintains a hierarchy of all three levels.

The most important plane for the organism is the mental–spiritual plane, which is the most central as well. A disturbance on this level is going to be felt acutely by the whole organism. Destruction of this level, the likes of which is witnessed during a severe mental disorder, takes away everything that is most important and precious to the individual, that which distinguishes him from the animals. Losing one's mental faculties is the worst thing that can happen to an individual. The organism, through its own physical structure, primarily protects this part and will not easily allow a disturbance to deeply penetrate it unless the organism has been greatly undermined.

The level next in importance is the emotional plane, and lastly comes the physical body. The organism will try to protect its innermost parts by stopping the disorder on more peripheral levels.

This idea of hierarchy is exemplified when we observe the evolution of a disease process within an individual. In the beginning the disease seems to be on the physical level, but if incorrect or suppressive treatment is applied, the disturbance leaves the physical body and proceeds to the innermost part of the human being. Then we start observing disturbances on the mental and emotional planes.

A woman with a vaginal discharge of any origin who applies local suppositories may suppress the discharge, however, she may soon develop more internal problems like insomnia and depression. But as soon as the discharge returns by either correct treatment or by sheer reaction of the defenses of the organism, the insomnia and depression go away. Witnessing such a case, which is frequent in women, we see the internalization of the disease, which is the "same" only in a different form, and which is more internal and therefore more painful and dangerous. Treatment has pushed the disease further inside and has actually broken the first line of defense that the organism had erected. The suppositories forcibly broke down the defenses, and that is why the organism put up a second line of defense, taking the form of sleeplessness and depression.

Of course, insomnia does not always show up after a vaginal discharge because the reaction will always be individual and will take the form to which each person is predisposed.

These reactions are not the usual side effects of drugs that we all know about, but are the combined inherent weaknesses of the organism that appear under the stress produced by the drugs. Another simple example of this process is the influence of antibiotics upon the ecology (microflora) of the intestines.

"Extended broad-spectrum antibiotic therapy is likely to induce candida due to disruption of the normal ecologic balance of the intestinal flora." [23]

"Antibiotics differ from the other drugs in that they not only exert a therapeutic effect but also alter the ecology of the microflora of the body and the environment. **Thus, antibiotic usage conjures up an image of fallout akin to that from a leaking nuclear reactor.**" [24]

The initial symptoms seem to disappear under the action of the medicine; in reality they are not cured but instead are pushed to deeper areas of the organism.

This concept is very important and has to be understood well from the very beginning: **Unless correct treatment is given, the seemingly curative action of the medicine may be suppressive.** It is around this concept that this treatise's whole argument about AIDS is based.

4. Each one of these planes is composed of multiple complex fields or organ systems that also maintain a hierarchical relationship.

In the same way that the three planes are in hierarchical importance, the systems or fields of energy or patterns within one plane are structured in a such a way that one system or organ has greater importance than another. For instance, a scratch on the brain will not have the same consequences that a scratch on the skin will have. Normally the consequences from a scratch on the brain are much more severe. That means that the brain is a much more important organ than the skin and therefore more protected, more guarded by the organism.

The whole organism is hierarchically organized, with some organs or biological systems being of greater or lesser importance than others and therefore enjoying a greater or lesser degree of protection.

This protection is afforded not only by the physical, anatomical position of an organ but also by the defense mechanism, a primary operant of the system. This defense mechanism includes the immune system as well as the reticuloendothelial, sympathetic, parasympathetic, hormonal and lymphatic systems. All these systems cooperate in producing a unique result; they maintain the homeostasis of *the organism* by keeping it in balance under all adverse conditions and, most of all, by protecting its vital and central organs.

For every drastic change, for every strong stress that is specific or non-specific, there is a mobilization of the defenses of the organism in order to maintain the optimum balance; or when the stress is too strong, the defense mechanism invokes "damage control," attempting to minimize the consequences of the assault. The main goal of the organism is to keep the disturbance as much to the periphery as possible.

Hierarchical Importance within the Physical Body

Just to provide a general idea, we shall list the organs according to their hierarchical importance in the system. This classification is not intended to be final in any way; it is only indicative and should be so taken by the reader. It is a very gross classification that can give the physician or healing practitioner an initial idea of the direction in which his treatment is going.

We begin with the physical body as the idea of hierarchy on this level is more easily understood and accepted. A gross enumeration of the main physical organs and systems is:

1. Central and peripheral nervous systems
2. Heart and vascular system
3. Pituitary and endocrine glands
4. Liver and digestive system
5. Lymphatic system
6. Lungs and respiratory system
7. Kidneys and urinary system
8. Testes/ovaries and genital system
9. Vertebrae and skeletal system
10. Muscular system
11. Mucous membranes
12. Skin

It must be understood that similar hierarchies exist within systems or organs. For example, certain areas of the brain are more vital than the peripheral nerve endings, etc.

While this classification may not be precise, it does provide a suitable frame of reference for understanding the concept of suppression. For example, if an individual suffers from a skin condition, eczema perhaps, which either of itself or as a consequence of suppressive treatment (e.g. cortisone ointment) disappears only to be succeeded by asthma (a lung condition), the person's health is deteriorating. His disease "condition" has moved in the wrong direction, more deeply within his body. Were the reverse to occur, the direction taken would be a curative one.

The same idea is valid for diseases that affect whole systems such as the nervous system, circulatory system, endocrine system, lymphatic system, digestive system, respiratory system, etc.

The same idea of hierarchy is also valid for the mental and emotional planes.

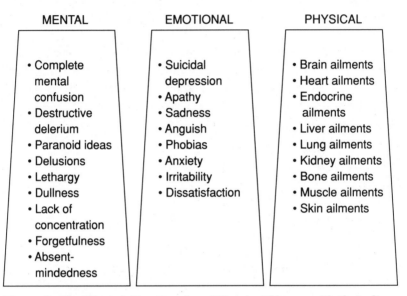

MENTAL	EMOTIONAL	PHYSICAL
• Complete mental confusion • Destructive delerium • Paranoid ideas • Delusions • Lethargy • Dullness • Lack of concentration • Forgetfulness • Absent-mindedness	• Suicidal depression • Apathy • Sadness • Anguish • Phobias • Anxiety • Irritability • Dissatisfaction	• Brain ailments • Heart ailments • Endocrine ailments • Liver ailments • Lung ailments • Kidney ailments • Bone ailments • Muscle ailments • Skin ailments

Figure 9: The Mental, Emotional and Physical Planes with their diverse systems classified in descending order of importance.

The argument here is that the mechanism that produces anxiety is a whole "system," like the circulatory or nervous system. In an individual a given stimulus could trigger either a centrally located or a more peripheral focus within the "anxiety system" of his psyche. A severe or mild anxiety syndrome could result in proportion to the depth of the irritated focus.

The same idea is valid for depression. A particular event can trigger either a severe depression that immediately leads to a suicidal impulse or a mild depression (which is dealt with much more easily than the former reaction). The phenomenon is similar to that seen in the nervous system. The effect would be quite different if a wound affected only peripheral nerve endings rather than the brain or central nervous system. But just as the systems themselves are classified according to their hierarchical importance, so are the different systems within each plane classified; e.g. the "irritability system," the "anxiety system," the "depression system," etc.

It is obviously better for a patient to be dissatisfied with something rather than be depressed; irritability is a better state than anguish; and anxiety is better than suicidal depression. The same thing applies to the mental level, as depicted in the diagram.

5. **Each of these three planes**—the mental, emotional and physical—though complex in nature, **constitute distinct and separate entities that differ essentially in their vibrational frequencies and informational patterns.** These three distinct planes interact with extreme intelligence and react to any stimulus in a concerted manner that is always consistent with their own idiosyncrasies.

It is obvious that mental energy is of a different vibrational frequency than emotional energy, or sexual energy, or physical energy. The quality of the energy used to move our hand is not the same as the quality of energy used to produce a thought. The energy that makes the heart pump is not of the same quality as the energy that produces an emotion. Different emotions have different qualities of energy as well. For example the quality of energy generated in a love situation is entirely different from that generated in a situation of anger or hatred. In short, the organism has the capacity to generate complex energy fields according to the information that has been engrafted in its internal codes (DNA, RNA, genes, chromosomes, etc.) through hereditary predisposition and personal experiences.

External, internal, positive or negative information can be received through any of these three planes, but the organism reacts to the information (stress) in a **total** and **individualistic** manner. For instance, an emotional shock that is received through the emotional plane is not always going to show a reaction on the emotional level. For example, a separation from a loved one that produces a shock which cannot be handled by the organism will tend to produce some type of reaction, which may be a skin eruption (skin), herpes on the lip (mucous membrane), a duodenal ulcer (digestive system), liver disturbance; anxiety, depression, suicidal depression (emotional level); mental confusion, delusions or paranoid ideation (mental level); or there may be some kind of effect on all of these levels. We see that the organism, according to the information inherent in its DNA, RNA, genes, chromosomes, etc., reacts in an entirely individualistic manner.

The same will apply for a shock received through the physical body (plane). These "shocks" can result from exposure to a virus, a bacteria, a very damp or otherwise adverse climate, etc. The organism will react to such a shock in a highly individualistic manner, distributing the final reaction to one, two or even all three planes. It is for this reason that massive treatments usually disappoint both their exponents and patients—because the results they produce are only on the material plane, therefore they are too "gross" and thus harmful, especially for sensitive organisms that do not possess a robust defense mechanism.

REFERENCES:

1. BATESON G: *Steps to an Ecology of Mind.* New York: Ballantine Books, 1972
2. CHAUCHARD P: *The Brain.* Translated by David Noakes. New York: Grove Press, 1962
3. KAMIYA J: Conscious control of brain waves. *Psychology Today 1968; 1: 57-60*
4. LYNN R: *Attention, Arousal and the Orienting Response.* Oxford: Pergamon Press, 1966
5. MUSES CM, YOUNG AM, eds: *Consciousness and Reality.* New York: Outer Bridge and Lazard, 1972
6. PELLETIER KR: Neurological substrates of consciousness. *J Altered States of Consciousness 197; 1: 2*
7. PELLETIER KR: Holistic applications of clinical biofeedback and meditation. *J Holistic Health 1976; 1*
8. PELLETIER KR: *Toward a Science of Consciousness.* New York: Random House, 1977
9. STEIN M, SCHIAVI RC, CAMERINO M: Influence of brain and behavior on the immune system. *Science 1976; 191: 435-440*
10. TUKE DH: *Illustrations of the influence of the mind upon the body in health and disease designed to eludidate the action of the imagination.* 2nd ed. London: J and A Churchill, 1884
11. WEIL A: *The Natural Mind.* Boston: Houghton Mifflin, 1973
12. BARBER T, DiCARA L, KAMIYA J, MILLER N, SHAPIRO D, STOYVA J: *Bio-feedback and Self-control: An Aldine Annual on the Regulation of Bodily Processes and Consciousness.* Chicago: Aldine-Atherton, 1970

13. BLUM GA: *Model of the Mind.* New York: Glencoe, 1968
14. FINGARETTE H: *The Self in Transformation: Psychoanalysis, Philosophy and the Life of Spirit.* New York: Basic Books, 1963
15. LUTHE W: Autogenic training: method, research, and application in psychiatry. *Dis Nerv Syst 1962; 23: 383*
16. VASILIEV L: *Experiments in Mental Suggestion.* Church Crookman, Hampshire, England: Institute for the Study of Mental Images, 1963
17. FERGUSON M: *The Brain Revolution.* Taplinger Publishing Company, 1973
18. MARTIN EW et al: *Hazards of Medication.* Toronto: JB Lippincott Co., 1971
19. SIMMONS HE: *An Overview of Public Policy and Infectious Diseases 1978; 89: 5 (part 2) 821-825*
20. *World Health Statistics Annual 1983*
21. *World Health Statistics Annual 1985*
22. *World Health Statistics Annual 1986*
23. HAROLD LC, BALDWIN RA: Ecologic effects of antibiotics. *FDA Papers 1967; 1: 20-24*
24. Antibiotic accountability. *N Engl J Med 1979; 301, 7: 380-381*

Chapter 5

DEFINITION AND MEASURE OF HEALTH

The first task of a science that claims its primary aim is to restore health should be to define what "health" is, what the target or goal of treatment is, and in what direction the patient should be guided during his treatment.

One should also define the parameters for measuring health. This should be defined so that anybody can easily ascertain whether an individual under treatment is progressing toward health or is actually regressing toward a deeper state of imbalance.

I doubt whether any medical graduate could provide these definitions; I also doubt that medical students are taught to recognize an ideal state of health or to identify the parameters that measure it.

When the pain is gone, when the inflammation has subsided, when a bothersome symptom has disappeared, when the pathology is no longer evident, the patient usually is pronounced cured. Yet there may be long-term disturbances caused by the treatment, especially in deeper or more subtle parts of the human organism such as the immune or hormonal systems or, even worse, in the mental or emotional planes, that are not taken into consideration. A treatment therefore should have a beneficial effect *simultaneously* on all these levels in order to claim that it is the right kind of treatment.

Treating the whole person, which is now accepted on a rhetorical level by everyone, should be more than a theoretical dictum; it should be an applied reality.

I hope to clearly show in this treatise that such an objective is almost impossible to attain through treatment with allopathic drugs, and that only through some form of alternative medicine practiced correctly, such as Homeopathy, Acupuncture, Osteopathy, Naturopathy, etc., can the potential for such a goal be realized.

The Definition of Health for the Physical Body

Disease, whether expressed through pain, discomfort or weakness, always tends to restrict the individual. Its opposite, health, gives a sense of freedom. This is the reason why in the definition that follows I have used the word "freedom" as a key word.

I also give a separate definition of health for each of the three planes since I know that an individual can be sick on one level while on another level he may appear completely healthy. For example, a schizophrenic that is deeply disturbed in his mental-emotional plane appears to be extremely healthy in his physical body. It is a well-established fact that severely mentally ill patients almost never get sick with physical ailments, even under the most adverse conditions, while others that suffer from physical ailments can be very healthy in their emotional and mental spheres.

As we have already stated, every pain, discomfort, uneasiness, distress or weakness of the physical body results in a limitation of freedom and a feeling of bondage to the pain or discomfort. The individual necessarily directs all his attention to the pain, to the exclusion of everything else, and of course loses his general sense of well-being. It is for this reason that health on the physical plane can be defined as follows: **Health is freedom from pain in the physical body, having attained a state of well-being.**

The Definition of Health on the Emotional Plane

On the emotional plane, that which enslaves the individual and absorbs all his attention is excessive passion—passion in the broadest sense and not with only a sensual connotation.

Excessive, inordinate passion for anything shows a degree of imbalance within the emotional plane. For instance, when an overwhelming erotic passion for another person reaches a point where murdering this person is contemplated because of jealousy, we definitely have a disease state rather than a love state. Passion for a cause, even a lofty one, that brings the individual to the point where he contemplates destructive actions against others is definitely a diseased state rather than justified idealism. A healthy state of the emotions never goes so far as to bring about destruction, but rather tries to follow the "golden mean" of the ancient Greeks.

Fanatical and dogmatic attitudes that divorce themselves from logic and understanding show a degree of unhealthy emotional involvement that usually results in some type of catastrophe, either for the individual or for others. Passionately loving somebody may mean that the degree of attachment is so great that if the love is not reciprocated, the individual may commit some kind of crime (homicide or suicide).

We too often mistake our emotional needs and insecurities for real love and affection. The latter two presuppose giving without reservation. It is emotional attachment that constantly makes demands of others under the pretense of giving. Certainly the opposite of passion—apathy—is no more desirable. Apathy is an extremely unhealthy emotional state, very much akin to the idea of death. What is desirable is a state of serenity and calm that is dynamic and creative, not passive, indifferent or destructive—a state where love and positive emotions prevail, as opposed to hatred and other negative emotions.

In order to justify their origin and destiny, human beings have to transcend their animal nature, and have to make **conscious efforts to evolve**, not so much in their physical body as in their mental and emotional spheres.

I believe that it is clear now that passion comes from weakness rather than strength on the emotional plane. Thus the definition for this plane should be: **Health on the emotional plane is freedom from passion, having as a result a dynamic state of serenity and calm.**

The Definition of Health on the Mental–Spiritual Level

To give a concise definition of health on the mental-spiritual plane is a rather difficult task because one must identify the most important mental-spiritual qualities, which if disturbed may seriously injure the mental equilibrium.

After much deliberation I have come to the conclusion that peace of mind can be drastically affected by egotism, selfishness and acquisitiveness. The more egotistical and selfish an individual is, the greater his potential for mental derangement.

It is a known fact that a person who is very egotistical can be quite upset when his authority, knowledge or attainments are challenged. A humble man with the same attainments will hardly react to the unjust criticism of others, and will actually see the positive side of the criticism and correct his course of action accordingly. The same "shocks" that can set off an egotist and destroy him can leave a humble man almost unaffected.

An egotistical industrialist who fails in his business and loses his factory cares more about the opinion that others now have of him than the fate of the families, including his own, that will have no means to support themselves. It is his ego that has been hurt. Even if he has plenty to live on without the factory, he will feel miserable after the failure and is bound to develop a host of symptoms because of his "false" and selfish grief.

In a similar way, acquisitiveness could become the core of mental disturbance. Can you imagine how an avaricious man might react to the loss of his physical wealth and the deep symptomatology that could result?

Hardly anyone today is totally free from the feelings of egotism, selfishness and acquisitiveness.

It is also a fact that the person engrossed in his own ego can neither see objectively nor perceive the truth. He thinks he always knows everything and knows it better than anyone else. Humanity has suffered great disasters because of such attitudes. Looking back in history we frequently recognize this quality and label it insanity.

We speak about the insanity of Hitler, Idi Amin Dada, even of the captain in charge of the *Titanic* whose arrogance cost the lives of hundreds. In our own way, every one of us is dealing with similar issues on a smaller scale. This "disease" called egotism and selfishness seems to be universal. That is why we are so likely to admire and worship the saints; we believe that they actually managed to subdue their egotism and sacrifice their own lives for the sake of others. We worship them as "superior" human beings because their accomplishment seems beyond our comprehension. Although rare, this "saint-like" attitude is the healthiest to possess; in such a state true peace of mind and happiness is achieved.

It is peculiar, though, that this state of health **can only be achieved through conscious efforts** of the individual, while the state of health of the physical body is a birthright.

There is a natural legacy and an inherent urge for human beings to evolve into people of "Love and Wisdom." Only then will there be hope for the human race. Not until we start seeing the issue in all of its dimensions will there be hope for a better state of health.

This imbalance we feel on the mental-spiritual plane is perhaps the most challenging and complicated issue we have to face. Nobody is exempt from this imbalance, though there are different degrees. The greater an individual's egotism and selfishness, the greater are his possibilities for a mental breakdown.

We can therefore define mental health as: **Freedom from selfishness in the mental sphere, having as a result total unification with Truth.**

So now we summarize the whole definition of Health: **Health is freedom from pain in the physical body, a state of well being; freedom from passion on the emotional plane, resulting in a dynamic state of serenity and calm; and freedom from selfishness in the mental sphere, having as a result total unification with Truth.** A truly healthy individual should therefore combine both divine qualities of Love and Wisdom.

It is obvious that such a state of health is an ideal and that nobody can possess it in its entirety; but the definition points to an ideal *Model* of health toward which therapeutic treatments should aspire. The more a patient under treatment approaches this state, the healthier he becomes; and the more he moves away from it, the less healthy he becomes.

The Measure of Health

It is obvious at this point that we need some parameters to measure health.

Some questions are required of us. For example: If we cure somebody of asthma and as a consequence he develops a heart condition, how do we know that this new state of health is better or worse than his previous condition? If we treat a patient with a cardiac condition and he improves, but after a certain period of time he develops a phobic state or an anxiety neurosis, can we say that the treatment benefited the patient?

We shall see that in order for a treatment to be successful it has to push the disorder's center of gravity more and more to the peripheral, the skin being the final avenue of expression, leaving the deepest parts of the human being—his mental and emotional levels—intact.

As I have said, the issue of determining an individual's exact degree of health is a complicated task requiring much research and involving a number of parameters before precise answers are possible. But as a general rule of thumb, we can say that a good parameter for measuring the health of an individual is the **degree to which he is free to create**. Anybody who is basically healthy will seek to create rather than destroy. By creativity, as I have stated previously, I mean all those actions that promote the interests and good of oneself and others. To the degree that one commits destructive acts toward either himself or others, the degree to which he is diseased is apparent.

THE RELATION OF THE HUMAN BEING WITH THE UNIVERSE

6. Man lives in the universe as an integral part of it. The individual actually exists and copes with the environment through his capacity to exchange energies with it.

Human beings are inseparably connected with their immediate and broader environment in different ways:

a. From food
b. From the air they inhale
c. From exposure to sunlight
d. From the earth's temperature
e. From exchanging energies with their universal environment

I do not believe anybody at the present time would dispute factors (a) through (d). What is perhaps still difficult to conceive is the notion that our existence depends entirely on our capacity to exchange energies with our environment at large, and that this exchange is absolutely necessary for the continuation of life on earth.

Although this aspect is extremely important for our existence and well-being, it has been entirely neglected in our search for health. I am sure everyone understands that in order for such energy exchanges to take place, we must have the necessary receptors, and they should be in good condition in order to do their fine and complex work.

A hypothetical question to ponder is: If in the research for therapeutic drugs this parameter is not taken into consideration, what will be the consequences for those receptors? When we ingest a chemical drug and we develop insomnia or some unexplained physical weakness, how much is this drug responsible for our insomnia? How much is it responsible for the blockage of the mechanisms and functions that replenish our energies during sleep?

We cannot afford to ignore such questions any longer because we will soon have to face the dire consequences of our voluntary "blindness."

7. It has yet to be recognized that information between the individual and his or her environment is communicated on an energy level through the smallest particle-energy bodies. These bodies contain a wealth of information and specific codes that can be decoded only by a "sympathetic" apparatus on a similar level.

Each one of us has an apparatus that receives and decodes cosmic energy waves carrying specific messages and serving. specific purposes, especially during our sleep state. Every night we, as energy systems, become receptive to an abundance of very valuable information in the form of dreams. Sleep and dreaming are absolutely necessary for the continuation of our existence and for inducing necessary "modifications." Let us give a simple example: During the waking state we are confronted with an emotional problem that we do not face properly but instead ignore, suppressing our emotional response. If that state is not corrected in one's sleep through "symbolic dreaming," it may remain to detrimentally affect one's health.

I understand that this concept is a bit abstract and difficult to support with scientific evidence. Nonetheless, here we are concerned with vital issues that touch upon life itself, and thus we cannot ignore certain facts that are of paramount importance for the understanding of our subject. Science, I am sure, will soon provide enough evidence to verify the existence of this kind of energy that permeates the cosmos and from which we draw reserves every night in order to continue living.

It is a well-known fact that we cannot live very long without sleep, especially certain stages, and it seems that sleep is even more important than food. What happens in our sleep that regenerates us to such an extent, and why is it that nothing else can replace this type of regeneration?

It seems that we live our lives on three different levels of existence:

a. The Subconscious, where the logical mind is afforded a secondary role, especially during sleep.
b. The Conscious, where the logical mind reigns completely during awake-time.
c. The Superconscious, where the logical mind has "calmed" down or has been completely silenced. This happens in rare moments during our awake-state or during deep states of contemplation.

It seems that the logical mind is not capable of sorting out all the messages and impressions it receives during its waking hours, and it needs sleep-time to clear up the "muddle" and undo the "jamming" that has taken place on a deeper level during the rest of the day. Dreams, whether they be symbolic, prophetic or completely meaningless to the logical mind, function to clear the basic ground for mental and emotional balance on a deeper subconscious level so that the individual can continue his life undisturbed. Dreams clear the "apparatus" so that "universal energy" will go through it without encountering "noise" or "jams" that accumulate during awake-time.

Some dreams may be understood by the logical mind, and this helps the individual understand some of his problematic issues on deeper levels. Some other dreams may appear meaningless or incomprehensible but still provide needed help on a subconscious level. Most of the time dreams originate from a certain kind of pathology, and their manifestation is an important aspect of the defense mechanism.

If the energy-receiving apparatus is damaged by a chronic disease, regeneration in sleep cannot take place easily and the individual will feel "unrefreshed" and constantly tired.

The most probable hypothesis regarding the sleep state is that we are "bathing in a pervasive sea of subtle energy." This kind of energy has been given different names by different people at various times in history. It has been called:

Prana by the Hindus,
Vis medicatrix naturae by Hippocrates,
Magnale by Paracelsus,
Alcahest by Van Helmont,
Astral light by the Kabbalists,

Azoth by the Alchemists,

Spiritus by Fludd,

Odic force by Reichenbach,

Animal magnetism by Mesmer,

Etheric energy or **bioenergy** or **simple substance** by occultists and metaphysicians like Swedenborg,

Vital energy or **vital force** or **vital body** by the vitalistic school,

Orgone by Reich,

Bioplasma by Russian researchers, etc.

The prospects are that we will probably hear it called by many different names in the future. For the sake of understanding in this treatise we shall call it **universal energy** because this more accurately identifies one of its main qualities—universality. I believe the most conclusive answer about this energy will soon be given by physicists who deal with "small clusters" (a new branch of physics that is rapidly developing).[1-7]

It appears that we are in constant communication with universal energy, continuously exchanging energies with it, especially under certain circumstances that will be explained.

As I have already mentioned, every night during sleep we "open up" to receive extremely valuable information. We receive this in the form of dreams and symbols[8-25] that are absolutely necessary for the continuation of life. It seems that it is not a haphazard energy but one of purpose, since it accomplishes specific things. From the vast reservoir of universal energy the individual organism draws a specific type of needed energy or information. This energy seems to bring about required corrections or rearrangements within the organism in order to allow the process of regeneration to occur.

As has been noted, a complete health science must take into account the content of and interrelations between the physical, emotional and mental planes of existence. In addition, the complex relationship of man with his environment demands attention in the healing arts. Consequently, any truly holistic approach to health should not only pay heed to the physical, mental and emotional planes, but should also consider:

1. The correct intake of nourishing, properly grown food (food quality, combination and quantity)

2. The correct method of breathing (respiratory habits and the control of air quality)

3. The possible need of correcting aberrant energy flow

REFERENCES:

1. FRIEDEL J: Small aggregates. *Helvetica Physica Acta 1983; 56: 507-520*

2. RAO BK, JENA P: Physics of small metal clusters: Topology, magnetism and electronic structure. *Physical Rev Bull 1985; 32(4): 2058-2069*

3. STEIN GD: Atoms and molecules in small aggregates. The fifth state of matter. *The Physics Teacher, November 1979; 603-613*

4. MUETTERTIES EL: Molecular Metal Clusters. *Science 1977; 196: 839*

5. ABRAHAM FF: *Homogenous Nucleation Theory.* New York: Academic Press, 1974

6. PAULING J, HUWARD R: *The Architecture of Molecules.* San Francisco: WH Freeman Co., 1964

7. MARTINS JL, BUTTET J, CAR R: Equilibrium geometries and electronic structures of small sodium clusters. *Physical Rev Let 1984; 53(7): 655-658*

8. FOULKES D, VOGEL G: Mental activity at sleep onset. *J Abnorm Psychology 1965; 70: 231-243*

9. BERGER R , OSTWALD I: Effects of sleep deprivation on behavior, subsequent sleep, and dreaming. *EEG Clin Neurophysiol 1962, 14, 297(b)*

10. CHERTOK L, KRAMARZ P: Hypnosis, sleep, and encephalography. *J Nerv Ment Dis 1959; 128: 227-238*

11. DEMENT W, KLEITMAN N: Cyclic variations in the EEG during sleep and their relation to eye movements, body motility, and dreaming *EEG Clin Neurophysiol 1957; 9: 637-690*

12. DeSANCTIS S, NEYROZ U: Experimental investigation concerning the depth of sleep. *Psych Rev 1902; 9: 254-282*

13. FOULKES D: Dreams report from different stages of sleep. *J Abnorm & Soc Psychol 1962; 65: 14-25*

14. FOULKES D: *The Physiology of Sleep.* New York: Scribners, 1966

15. FOULKES D: Theories of dream formation and the recent studies of sleep consciousness. *Psych Bull 1964; 62: 236-247*

16. FOULKES D, SPEAR P, SYMONDS J: Individual differences in mental activity at sleep onset. *J Abnorm Psychol 1966; 71: 280-286*

17. GOODENBOUGH D, LEWIS H, SHAPIRO A, JARET L, SLECER I: Dream reporting following abrupt and gradual awakening from different types of sleep. *J Pers Soc Psychol 1965; 2: 170-179*

18. KALES A: *Sleep: Physiology and Pathology.* Philadelphia: Lippincott, 1969

19. KETY S, EVARTS E, WILLIAMS H: *Sleep and Altered States of Consciousness.* Baltimore: Williams & Wilkins, 1967

20. KNIPPNER S, HUGHES W: Dreams and human potential. *J Human Psychol 1970; 10, (1), 1-20*

21. LUBY E, FROHMAN C, GRISSEL J, LENZO J, GOTTLIEB J: Sleep deprivation: effects on behavior, thinking, motor performance, and biological energy transfer systems. *Psychosom Med 1960; 22: 182-192*

22. OSWALD I: *Sleeping and Waking: Physiology and Psychology.* New York: Elsevier, 1962

23. RECHTSCAFFEN A, VERDONE P, WHEATON J: Reports of mental activity during sleep. *Canad Psychiat Assn J 1963; 8: 400-414*

24. RECHTSCAFFEN A, VOGEL G, SHAIKUN G: Interrelatedness of mental activity during sleep. *Arch Gen Psychiat 1963; 9: 536*

25. WILLIAMS R, WEBB W: *Sleep Therapy: A Bibliography and Commentary.* Springfield, Ill: Charles C Thomas, 1966

Chapter 7

DISSOCIATION OF THE LEVELS

As we have already tried to show, the *Model* presented here deals mostly with the energy complex of the human organism and considers it the foundation on which the organism is built and therefore of primary importance. We shall now proceed a step further and state that the mental and emotional planes not only constitute distinct entities, but also "dissociate" from the physical body under certain conditions.

This is an issue that if proven true would confirm the independence of the different levels as well as their distinct energy structures.

8. All evidence permits us to assume that there is not only a possibility but a necessity, under certain circumstances, for the organism to "unite" or "dissociate" the complex energy fields of the mental-emotional planes, or parts thereof, and the fields of the physical body.

A human being is actually an energy unit that can generate or receive energy. To become receptive to this energy, the mental-emotional parts must dissociate, to a certain degree, from the physical. This could be an issue for dispute, but new evidence is providing more than enough information to overcome scepticism.

There are several circumstances under which we witness such a phenomenon:

a. Sleep
b. Somnambulism
c. Fainting
d. Surgical anesthesia
e. Hypnosis
f. Yogic and religious trances
g. Schizophrenia

h. Chemically induced dissociation through hallucinogenic drugs

i. Apparent death

a. Sleep

During sleep we do essentially nothing. We lie down, close our eyes and drift into oblivion. Not surprisingly, as healthy individuals, we wake up in the morning fully rested and refreshed with much more energy than before going to bed. Now just where did this energy come from? The most probable hypothesis is that it came from an energy source and that the organism had the capacity to tap this energy source.

In order that regeneration be full, the dissociation of the finer from the grosser elements of the organism should be as complete as possible. That is why we may have different kinds of sleep with different states of regeneration. An obvious approach for assessing the functions of sleep is to prevent its occurrence and search for resulting consequences. Through different sleep experiments scientists have assessed that there are two states of sleep, called NREM (non-rapid eye movement) and REM (rapid eye movement). NREM sleep contains four stages, of which the fourth stage is that characterized by Delta waves and the highest threshold to arousal. In other words, in this stage the person is in deep sleep, and it is very difficult to awaken him. After this fourth stage of NREM sleep the person goes into REM sleep. This neurophysiological explanation is somewhat analogous to the situation I am talking about concerning the different degrees of dissociation and regeneration occurring in the different stages of sleep.

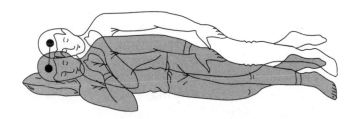

Figure 10: First phase of sleep: The dissociation is not complete.

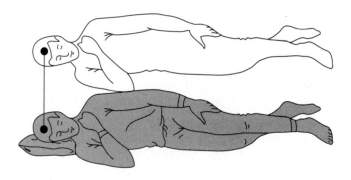

Figure 11: Second phase: Deeper sleep.

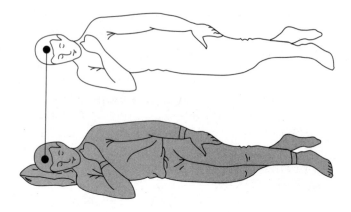

Figure 12: Third phase: Very deep sleep.

As shown in the accompanying diagrams, during phase one the dissociation is not complete, and the individual in this condition will experience only partial regeneration. During this phase the individual will have some awareness of what is going on in the environment. We observe this in someone who is "half asleep"—his mind is somewhat working together, as is his hearing. This individual is not really letting go of the physical world and so is not fully regenerating. Therefore, he will not rise from his half-sleep completely refreshed.

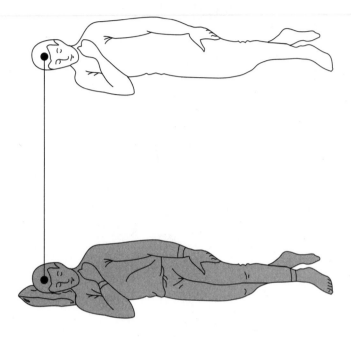

Figure 13: Fourth phase: The deepest state of sleep, where the dissociation is great and there is usually difficulty in reconnecting.

In the second phase the individual goes deeper into sleep and the dream phase begins. The regeneration in this phase is much better. His conscious mind cannot easily become aware of the physical world, and it is more difficult to hear sounds in the environment, but he still can be easily aroused.

In the third phase he is deep into "oblivion." This is deep sleep and he cannot be awakened easily. Regeneration is fairly complete in this phase. During one night's sleep, an individual goes in and out of these stages according to the needs of his organism.

There is a fourth stage of sleep that is the deepest and most dissociated of all. This is the stage which the organism needs the most in order to regenerate.[1,2]

b. Somnambulism (sleepwalking)

In this condition, individuals sit up in bed, walk or carry out automatic and semi-purposeful complex motor activities. Patients remain unconscious and will resist being aroused.

Somnambulism is a pathological state where the interacting fields are confused and the physical body is perplexed. But regeneration can take place because the conscious mind together with the five senses are being "silenced."

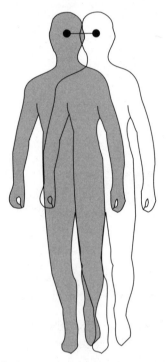

Figure 14: Somnambulism.

c. Fainting

In this phenomenon we witness an ultimate reaction of the defenses to save the organism from extreme danger. The finer elements of the organism containing the higher faculties and senses are deeply dissociated from the grosser elements to the extent that nothing is felt, even if there is extreme pain, as in the case of an amputation.

In this situation we witness the effort of the organism to protect the whole system from the repercussions of extreme pain, which could have a fatal effect upon the heart or brain. Again, at this point we observe in the organism the same principle of "knocking out" the conscious mind, feelings and five senses.

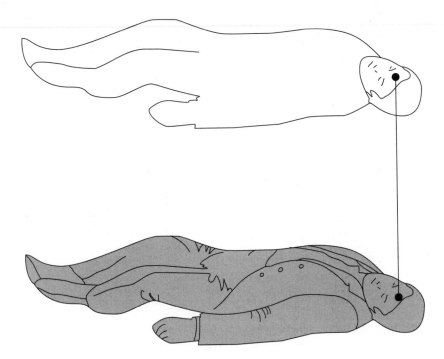

Figure 15: Fainting.

d. Surgical anesthesia

With surgical anesthesia we witness the exteriorization of the finer levels of the organism, quite similar to what we witness in fainting. Many times we hear of strange phenomena in both of these categories. People are aware of being out of their bodies and watch their physical form lying on the operating table or on the ground; they may even hear the conversation of others in the vicinity. These testimonies once again confirm the theories expounded in this treatise. Such experiences have been reported again and again during comatose states or "pre-death" situations.

For an example of a drug experience, James cites Symond's description of undergoing chloroform anesthesia:

"....I thought that I was near death; when suddenly, my soul became aware of God, who was manifestly dealing with me, handling me." [3-5]

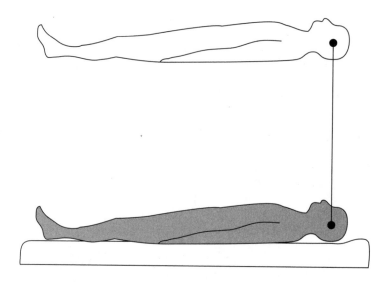

Figure 16: Surgical anesthesia.

e. Hypnosis

During hypnosis the subject experiences a dissociation of mental and physical planes and loses control of his rational mind. The hypnotist can manipulate the mind, feelings and senses of the subject through a specialized technique.

What is important and interesting to observe is how many different possibilities the organism has at its disposal to associate these finer elements with and dissociate them from the grosser ones. Research in these areas may reveal very interesting phenomena in connection with the genesis of diseases in general and may lend strength to the notion that there is a need for more refined therapeutic tools than the crude drugs being used today by allopathic medicine.[6-13]

f. Yogic and religious trances

There are many reports about yogis, especially from India, who remain in trance for days. They go "outside" of their body, yet at the same time their physical body remains entirely rigid. Of course, such states are extremely regenerating but very difficult for ordinary people to attain. Such trances are actively and consciously brought about by yogis or other religious adepts. In other words, the individual by himself severs his connection with the physical-material world. There are so many accounts of such incidents that the concept does not require further documentation.[14-24]

In such cases, according to the principle that **similars attract similars,** the purity, clarity and coherence of the field of the individual will determine the quality (higher or lower regions) of the universal energy with which he will come into contact. In this kind of dissociation the individual relinquishes conscious control over his physical body and opens his being to the influence of the cosmic (universal) fields that are most similar to his in vibrational quality or frequency.

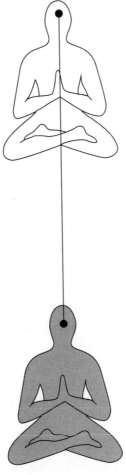

Figure 17: Yogic states: The body is immobilized and the five senses completely cut off.

g. Schizophrenia

In this disease, like so many other psychotic disorders, the patient is living in a condition of partial exteriorization (dissociation), somewhere between the physical world and dream world. He is able to receive impressions from both spheres at the same time. It is interesting to note that the word schizophrenia, which comes from Greek, literally means a split or disconnection of the mind. What is of great importance is that chemical drugs can induce such states; witness the effects of hallucinogenic drugs.[25-29]

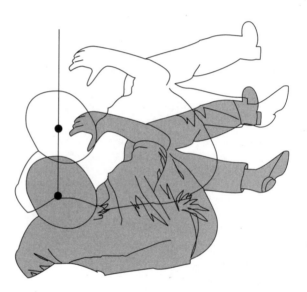

Figure 18: Schizophrenic state: Hallucination.

h. Chemically induced "dissociation" using hallucinogenic drugs

This is certainly a well-known and thoroughly documented phenomenon.[6,12, 30-48] In this condition, those that ingest the hallucinogen are known to exist for hours or even days in a state of "dissociation." In this state, the drugged person perceives other ethereal worlds, often losing the ability to discern the objective realities of this physical world.

Sometimes there is a partial dissociation experienced under the influence of these drugs. This is also seen in schizophrenia, where people live in their own fantasy world and have a confused perception of reality and the physical world.

i. Apparent death

Here we witness the longest and deepest dissociation that can exist while the organism is still alive. This state can be viewed as existing on the threshold between life and death. The person appears to be in a state that is very similar to death, yet he will snap out of this state in a few hours or a few days. What is it that returns? What was missing during this time of apparent death? Were the mental-emotional planes at all times residing with the five senses? These are some legitimate questions one has to ask about such phenomena. Dr. Elizabeth Kubler-Ross[3] has devoted her life to examining this and similar phenomena of "near-death" experiences and has presented her message to the whole medical profession. The message is that there is definitely something else that exists beyond the physical body.

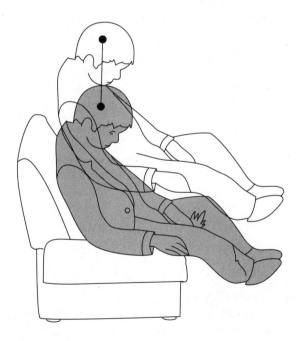

Figure 19: A subject under the influence of hallucinogenic drugs perceives images of another dimension.

The phenomena enumerated so far have certain common factors:

1. Temporary suspension of the logical mind (part or parts of the mental level)
2. Temporary suspension of feelings (either part or all of the emotional level)
3. Temporary suspension of the five senses (part or whole)

These phenomena can take place because the human organism has a structure that is not a pure physical form but is also an energy form. Some like to call it the "ethereal body," others the "astral body," still others "bioenergy"; while physicists formerly called it anti-matter, and those currently doing research on "small clusters" like to call it a "fifth state of matter." We do not care what it is called, as long as everyone understands and acknowledges that this state of matter has "new qualities" that very much resemble the qualities of energy.

The age-old disputes between the materialists (believers in only the purely physical world) and those contemptuously called "metaphysicians" have cost humanity a lot of suffering. We hope this will come to an end soon for the benefit of humanity.

It is time that we unify and utilize the totality of human knowledge in all its diverse manifestations—the scientific, the philosophical, the religious and the metaphysical.

Not only must we integrate these factors, but we have to do it as quickly as possible. Scientists have to learn to listen to philosophers as well as religious advocates and metaphysicians, while philosophers and metaphysicians have to integrate the findings of science in their philosophical contemplation. There will be hope for this planet only if a new type of individual emerges who will integrate the knowledge of the human mind bequeathed to us by centuries of effort and suffering.

9. The different degrees of dissociation possible indicate the extreme complexity of the fields generated by the human body and the sophisticated interconnections that give forth such variable phenomena.

It is interesting to observe that a dissociation occurs in many more situations than have been enumerated. For instance, when somebody concentrates on solving a problem he uses a certain degree of dissociation to isolate himself from environmental distractions. In such cases it is normal for him to be unaware of a nearby noise or another person entering the room, although his eyes are open.

In order to do abstract thinking, we have to dissociate from the environment. Everyone has probably had the experience of infuriating a wife or husband because you did not pay attention to what she or he was saying. You did not hear them, not because you did not care, but because you did not hear it while you were absorbed in your own thoughts. You were dissociated to a certain degree.

So, what we see from all these examples is that there are levels of existence which are part of the human entity but have a separate existence from the physical body.

10. "Dissociation" is essential for the continuation of life.

When the physical body is no longer fit to continue its function, being very tired, exhausted or badly hurt, dissociation is absolutely necessary in order to prevent further deterioration.

It is only during such a state that the flow of energy necessary for the regeneration of the individual can take place. The process should occur in a natural way, free from the effects of chemical stimulation.

A capacity to disconnect **at will** presupposes a high degree of evolution of the individual and gives him the possibility to regenerate at will.

For regeneration to take place, the conscious mind together with the five physical senses has to be subdued in **a natural way**; e.g. sleep, concentration states, self-hypnosis, meditational states, ecstasy states, deep religious experiences, yogic exteriorizations, etc. In other words, the individual has to cut his connection with the physical world.

During the process of dissociation, the normal individual, having lost control over his physical body, opens his being to the influence of the cosmic (universal) fields of energy that are **most similar** to the vibrational frequencies of his own fields. This is the reason that different people have different experiences during such states, some very frightening and others very pleasant.

It should be noted that the youth of today and of recent decades have, with desperation and great zeal, been attempting to acquire the ability to exteriorize from their bodies. In trying to achieve this they have used hallucinogenic drugs, taken up the practice and study of Eastern philosophies, and adopted new ways of life. Such youths usually seek spiritual or mystical experiences.

The use of hallucinogenic agents has been known since ancient times, but it was closely related to mystical or religious ceremonies. The initiates of ancient countries like Greece, Egypt and India used specific people who were gifted with a sensitivity or a "sixth" sense. Under the spell of a mystical ceremony aided by specific drugs, these people were in a position to unravel mysteries and foresee future events or situations.

The use of such agents in our modern time has little to do with such mystical experiences, and many youths experience an amplification of their own subconscious fears or desires rather than objective truth or future events. As a consequence of this "unreasonable" approach, the results are either insignificant or disastrous. Very frightening experiences often result from careless experimentation with drugs. Many times the negative results of these "trips" remain for life.

Aside from using chemical means to achieve dissociation of mind and body, there are mental and spiritual exercises that can give the practitioner a sense of "peace of mind" together with a sense of "regeneration." All these so-called esoteric or mystical practices, originating primarily in the East, base their success on a simple fact—that if the logical mind is silenced enough, or completely stopped in its activity, a sense of deep peace and regeneration ensues.

It has to be clarified that spiritual or mystical experiences cannot be the result of forcefully induced conditions but are rather the culmination of mature and continuous spiritual efforts.

In order to attain a permanent state of "altered consciousness" the individual has to overcome certain automatic behavioral patterns and mind conditioning, requiring a "super" effort on the part of the individual. The attainment of a temporary state of "altered consciousness" can many times be accomplished by meditation, prayer, contemplation, drugs, etc. All such experiences point to the fact that the human organism is possessed with an infinite potential for regeneration and spiritual evolution. However, the "unauthorized" entrance into such realms always holds unpleasant surprises for the intruder, somewhat the same way one feels when entangled in a nightmare.

As mentioned, the purity, clarity and coherence of the energy fields of the individual will determine the quality of the "cosmic energy" with which he will come in contact. To further clarify this issue, we can say that the etheric body (energy fields) of each individual is not totally positive or totally negative, but is a mixture of the two, and thus the degree of clarity or in religious terms, the degree of purity, is always relative, never absolute. No one is absolutely pure or absolutely evil. There are only relative degrees of purity or impurity just as there are relative degrees of health and disease. So, simplistic as it may sound, the purer a person is at a given moment, the more pleasant and regenerating the experience of dissociation.

As an example, let us say that you went through a religious experience at confession. In utter sincerity you confessed everything that was burdening your soul, and you came out rejuvenated and happy. If at this moment of maximum purity you have an experience of dissociation, then it is going to be a very pleasant one.

Later on, you again accumulate some bad experiences. You commit transgressions, acts that you consider immoral, unethical and evil. Following these acts the situation arises where you, the same individual, will have a much different, more negative experience during dissociation, as this experience will be affected to a great degree by the relative impurity of the moment. Your reality at the moment will affect the result; if this reality is negative, containing transgressions against yourself and others, so will your dissociation experience be negative.

REFERENCES:

1. ANGREW H, WEBB W, WILLIAMS R: The effects of stage four sleep deprivation. *EEG Clin Neurophysiol 1964; 17: 68-70*
2. FOULKES D, VOGEL G: Mental activity at sleep onset. *J Abnorm Psych 1965; 70: 231-243*
3. KUBLER-ROSS E
4. MONROE R: *Journeys Out of the Body*. Garden City, New York: Doubleday & Co., 1971

5. TART C: A second psychophysiological out-of-the-body experience in a gifted subject. *Int J Parapsychol 1967; 9: 251-258*
6. AARONSON B: Hypnosis, depth perception and schizophrenia. *Paper, Eastern Psych Assn, Philadelphia, PA; 1964*
7. BEERS C: *A Mind that Found Itself.* New York: Atherton Press, 1965
8. HUXLEY A: *The Doors of Perception.* New York: Harper & Bros., 1954
9. LEVINE J, LUDWIG A: Alterations of consciousness produced by combination of LSD, hypnosis, and psychotherapy. *Psychopharm 1965; 7: 123-217*
10. LUDWIG A, LEVINE J: Alterations of consciousness produced by hypnosis. *J Nerv Ment Dis 1965; 140, 146-153*
11. MOSS C: *The Hypnotic Investigation of Dreams.* New York: John Wiley & Sons, 1967
12. SHOR R, ORNE E: *The Nature of Hypnosis: Selected Basic Readings.* New York: Holt, Rhinehart & Winston, 1965
13. TART C: Hypnosis suggestion as a technique for the control of dreaming. Paper. *Amer Psychol Bull 1965; 63, 87-99*
14. YOGANANDA PARAMAHANSA: *The Autobiography of a Yogi.* Encinitas, CA: Self-Realization Fellowship, 1954
15. GODNEY K: An examination into physiological changes alleged to take place during the trance state. *Proc Soc Psych Res 1938-1939; 45, 43-68*
16. KASAMATSU A, HIRAI T: Science of Zazen. *Psychologia 1963; 6, 86-91*
17. KASAMATSU A, SHIMAZONO Y: Clinical concept and neurophysiological basis of the disturbance of consciousness. *Psychiat Neuro Jap 1957; 11: 969-999*
18. KNOWLES D: *The English Mystical Tradition.* London: Burnes & Oates, 1961; 57
19. MAHARISHI MAHESH YOGI: *The Science of Being and the Art of Living.* Available through local branches of Students International Meditation Society in most large cities, 1966
20. STACE W: *Mysticism and Philosophy.* Philadelphia & New York: JB Lippincott, 1960
21. WENGER M, BAGHI B: Studies of autonomic function in practitioners of Yoga in India. *Behav Science 1961; 6: 312-323*
22. WENGER M, BAGHI B, ANAND B: Experiments in India on "voluntary" control of the heart and the pulse. *Circulation 1961; 24: 1319-1325*
23. WOODS J: *The Yoga-system of Patanjali.* Harvard Oriental series. Cambridge, Mass: Harvard University Press, 1914; 42
24. BRUNTON P: *A Search in Secret India.* B. I. Publications, 1970
25. De VITO R, FRANK I: Ditran: searchlights on psychosis. *J Neuropsychiat 1964; 5: 300-305*
26. GREIFENSTEIN R, De VAULT M, YOSHITAKE J, GAJEWSKI E: A study of L-arylocyclohixylamine for anesthesia. *Anesthes & Anelges 1958; 37: 283-294*
27. LAWES T: Schizophrenia, "sernyl" and sensory deprivation. *Brit J Psychiat 1963, 109: 243-250*
28. ENGLE G, ROMANO J: Delirium: a syndrome of cerebral insufficiency. *J Chron Dis 1959; 24: 691-697*

29. CHRISTIANSON G, KARLSSON B: Sniffing: a means of intoxication among children. *Svenska Lakartindigen 1957; 54: 33-44*
30. BAN T, LOHRENZ Z, LEHMANN H: Observations on the action of Sernyl—a new psychotropic drug. *Canad Psych Assn J 1961; 6: 150-157*
31. BERLIN L, GUTHRIE T, WEIDER A, GOODELL H, WOLFF H: Studies in human cerebral function: the effects of mescaline and lysergic acid on cerebral process pertinent to creative activity. *J Nerv Ment Dis 1955; 122: 487-491*
32. COHEN S: LSD and the anguish of dying. *Harper's Magazine 1965; 231: 60-72, 77-78*
33. COHEN S, SILVERMAN A, SHMAVONIAN B: Psychophysiological studies in altered sensory environments. *J Psychosom Res., 1962; 6: 259-281*
34. CROCKET R, SANDISON R, WALK A: *Hallucinogenic Drugs and their Psychotherapeutic Use.* London: JQ Lewis, 1963
35. De ROPP R: *Drugs and the Mind.* New York: Grove Press, 1957
36. FISHER R: *Origin and Mechanisms of Hallucination.* New York: Plenum Press, 1970
37. HOROWITZ M: The imagery of visual hallucinations. *J Nerv Ment Dis 1964; 138: 513-523*
38. MALITZ S, ESECOVER H, WILKENS B, HOCH P: Some observations on psylocybin, a new hallucinogen, in volunteer subjects. *Comp Psychiat 1960; 1: 8-17*
39. MASTERS R, HOUSTON J: *The Varieties of Psychedelic Experience.* New York: Holt, Rhinehart & Winston, 1966
40. McGLOTHIN W, CIHEN S, McGLOTHIN M: Long-lasting effects of LSD on normals. *Los Angeles: Institute of Government and Public Affairs, 1967*
41. OSMOND H: A review of the clinical effects of psychomimetic agents. *Ann NY Acad Sci 1957; 66(3): 418-434*
42. OSTER G: *The Science of Moire Patterns.* Barrington, NJ: Edmund Scientific Co., 1964
43. OSTFELD A: Effects of LSD-25 and JB-388 on tests of visual and perceptual function in man. *Fed Proc 1961; 20: 866-883*
44. PAHNKE H: *Drugs and Mysticism: An Analysis of the Relationship between Psychedelic Drugs and the Mystical Consciousness.* Cambridge, Mass: Harvard University, 1963
45. SAVAGE C: Variations in ego feelings induced by LSD-25. *Psychoanal Rev 1955; 42: 1-16*
46. SOLOMON D: *LSD: The Consciousness-expanding Drug.* New York: GP Putnam & Sons, 1964
47. WHITMAN R, PIERCE C, MAAS J: *Drugs and Dreams.* In L Uhr & J Miller, *Drugs and Behavior.* New York: John Wiley & Sons, 1960; 591-595
48. TART CT: *Altered States of Consciousness.* New York: John Wiley & Sons, 1969

Chapter 8

EVOLUTION OR DEGENERATION

**11. The human being must be understood as a very
complex energy unit with the potential for either
evolution or *degeneration*.**

By **evolution** we mean a greater degree of coherence in
informational patterns leading to an enhanced capacity for
creativity and **longevity.**

By **degeneration** we mean a greater degree of confusion in
these informational patterns with an increased tendency for
destruction.

Every human being has the potential to be more cohesive,
complete and organized and therefore to progress toward regeneration. But at the same time the potential exists for him to be
adversely affected by different external or internal negative
factors that can disrupt and provoke the degeneration of his
whole system.

That which evolves or degenerates is not only the material
body but the emotional and spiritual aspects of the human
being. These two aspects (the material and the spiritual-psychic) may not coincide in their progression or regression. In
other words, while the physical body may be degenerating, the
mental level—and especially the spiritual aspect of that level—
may progress to a greater degree of coherence or vice-versa. For
example, during a period when the physical body may be badly
afflicted by a severe chronic disease, the psychic-spiritual
planes of this human being may progress to greater degrees of
organization and coherence. We have examples of geniuses
whose capacity for scientific or artistic achievement was great at
a time when their physical bodies were degenerating from a
chronic disease. It is also not accidental that many times we
witness a strange phenomenon in those who are dying from
severe afflictions. At this time they put their best selves forward,
showing a strong spiritual turn of mind and a loving disposition

not previously exhibited in their life when they were considered "healthy."

We may also witness the opposite—mentally ill people exhibit a tremendous resilience in their physical bodies; they seldom get sick, even when subjected to severely hazardous situations. Unlike "healthy" children, autistic children seldom get sick with acute or infectious diseases. It is a well-established fact that severely mentally ill patients in psychiatric wards seldom suffer from infections despite exposure to very adverse conditions, especially in underdeveloped countries. This happens because the center of gravity of the disturbance is primarily concentrated in the deeper planes of existence, leaving the physical body intact.

This observation, although extremely important, has not been fully understood or appreciated even by those who are quite experienced in dealing with alternative methods of therapy.

This irregular and uncoordinated development of the human being, each level progressing or regressing separately instead of uniformly as one might expect, is largely an effect of prevailing sociocultural norms. So often the pressures of society seem to coerce the individual into adopting unhealthy and at times devious courses of action. There are myriad ways that the human mind has devised to silence or even "kill" the emotions. This is done systematically in western societies where phrases are heard such as, "You should never show your emotions," "Don't be so emotional," and "If you cry you are weak and a nuisance to others."

Another disastrous practice that has taken place, especially among many of today's youth, is that by separating their emotions from their physical body many have pursued the path of hedonism instead of love. In choosing sex over love they have chosen a path with consequences so subtle and deeply disastrous that they will probably feel the effects for the rest of their lives.

Instead of really falling in love such that the sexual act becomes the culmination of a regenerative and deeply satisfying process, they opt for the physical "orgasm," divorced from any emotional investment—a choice that robs them of far more precious, creative and subtle energies. They are left with an indescribable emptiness, a depletion of energy and an emotional "sclerosis" that makes them look old and emotionally dead, even at the age of 25.

The misunderstanding or lack of understanding of the function and importance of the emotional plane is due to the fact that it is the most potent generator of human pain and suffering. By killing this side of their nature, some people think they can avoid pain.

Few understand the meaning of such pain and the potential it contains for the evolution of the human species. Few understand that it is exactly this kind of suffering, coming from this plane, that bestows a quality that distinguishes us from an otherwise completely animalistic and crude existence. Few take into consideration the important role of the emotions, especially people in established medicine. When these emotions become extreme, they are deadened with strong chemical drugs. The price we shall have to pay in the near future for such unwise practices may be so high that it will border on the disastrous. Emotionally hard, sick and devious people will inflict horror and pain on each other without the normal restraints imposed by a "good and kind heart." Health practitioners, more than anyone else, should understand and utilize such knowledge in a correct manner.

Chapter 9

STIMULUS OR INFORMATION

**12. The organism always reacts as a totality to any given
stimulus. In its natural condition, the organism recognizes a stimulus as information to which it is
susceptible, and thereby vulnerable; this susceptibility generates an attraction and responsiveness to
the stimulus.**

Stimuli can be specific like bacteria, microbes, viruses, fungi,
etc., or non-specific like climatic changes, emotional grief,
mental upsets, shocks, etc.

An organism will be affected only by those stimuli to which it
is predisposed and to which it has a particular affinity; this will
be called its susceptibility. All other stimuli will leave it unaffected or unharmed.

Susceptibility to certain stimuli has to be understood as a
potentially precarious state of health which the organism has
had since birth or has developed after certain specific stresses.
At a certain point in time and while the organism is under stress,
this susceptibility to certain stimuli unfolds into an actual
pathological condition (into an acute or chronic disease). These
reactions (symptoms of diseases) are needed by the organism in
order to counteract the stress. This unfolding is a natural
process that springs from the law of selection, which states that
if the individual is strong enough, he will survive the crisis and
will come out of it deeply "cleansed" and even stronger.

The situation is entirely different if the organism is assaulted
by a powerful drug that is introduced into it (especially on a long-
term basis). These prescription and non-prescription drugs that
are ingested every day by millions of people (patients, drug
addicts, etc.) throughout the world have an unlimited power to
destroy the defenses of the human organism, especially its
immune system. AIDS, Chronic Fatigue Immune Dysfunction
Syndrome (CFIDS), candida, cancer, schizophrenia, arthritis,

arteriosclerosis, Alzheimer's dementia and other chronic degenerative diseases are a few examples of the consequences of such violations of the body's ecology.

13. **The power of the stimulus (or information) is directly proportional to the organism's degree of susceptibility (or vulnerability) to it.**

Different organisms have varied degrees of sensitivity or vulnerability to different stresses. For instance, an organism with a great sensitivity to a specific bacterium or virus will, upon coming into contact with that microorganism, react immediately and dramatically with severe symptomatology. The more susceptible the organism is, the more drastic and immediate is the reaction, and therefore the more dangerous the outcome of the disease. Another person who is not susceptible to the same virus can literally consume it without any effect. This is perfectly exemplified in the incident involving Professor Petenkoffer, M.D., and Dr. Koch, who discovered the Tb bacillus. Professor Petenkoffer, in order to prove to his colleagues and Koch that it was not only a microbe that was needed to initiate a certain disease but also the organism's susceptibility or predisposition, drank a vial containing the Tb bacillus. He literally ingested the microbe but suffered no ill effects from it.

A man receives an emotional shock when a friend informs him that his wife is having an extramarital affair. Because of a similar previous experience during his first marriage, the man has been sensitized to such information. He therefore has a predisposition to be greatly affected by such negative stress, and his organism undergoes devastating consequences: he develops depression, a heart attack, diabetes or a terrible skin reaction, the exact nature of the reaction depending upon the predispositions inherent in his genetic make-up.

A person who is sensitive to rose pollen will have devastating effects when coming in contact with it, while others will enjoy the roses' fragrance.

Patient A is very sensitive to a certain antibiotic and literally falls apart upon contact with a small quantity of it. The allergic reactions (hypersensitivity) provoked by even an infinitesimal amount of penicillin and its derivatives are already well known.[1-4] Patient B can withstand considerable quantities of the same antibiotic without adverse effects.

Some people who take an antibiotic won't develop a disease or serious side effects immediately, but will have delayed hypersensitivity. If we keep on giving the drug in an unwise way, it is certain to cause a predisposition even in those who initially were not sensitive to it. Recently a lot of interest has been focused upon delayed hypersensitivity caused by antibiotics such as rifampin, amphotericin B, metrodinoxazole, doxycycline and tetracycline.[5-7]

In my opinion, antibiotics that could have been life-saving and a blessing in really dangerous cases are prescribed in such a way that they will prove to be one of the greatest curses of our modern civilization. They may spare a patient's life but leave him blind, deaf, afflicted with kidney, liver or brain damage, bone necrosis, ulceration of the bowel, intestinal hemorrhage, skin scars, extreme sensitivity to sunlight, or other disabilities that may last for months or years. Only during the past decade have we begun to recognize the magnitude, severity and complexity of the problem. Today it is only too obvious that adverse drug reactions represent a major public health menace of alarming proportions.[8] Accordingly, I conclude that antibiotics should be given only in emergency situations and only if the life of a patient is threatened.

14. Stimuli or information can be positive or negative, promoting either evolution or degeneration.

We all know the beneficial effect of providing insight or information to people, especially when it concerns the "gray" or confused areas of their emotional or mental spheres. The whole idea of psychotherapy is based on this assumption. In the same way, a medicinal plant or mineral has to provide this much-needed information to really benefit the human organism.

Once the stimulus (which should always be understood as a subtle energy charge) passes a critical level (the organism's ability to automatically cope with it), a change takes place where self-regulation or disturbance occurs, which is akin to the nature of a **quantum jump** evoking a new rearrangement of energy patterns. By this quantum jump we imply that the organism, in a split second, changes its level of health; it marks the beginning of evolutionary or degenerative processes. This jump becomes necessary for the organism to cope with the new situation created by a hostile or a positive stimulus.

Hostile stimuli are comprised not only of bacteria and viruses, but also chemical drugs (medicines). The human organism when confronted with a drug initially attempts to eradicate the drug's toxic effects, and so re-establish order. However, when exposed to a frequently recurring onslaught of drugs, things take a different turn. A primary example would be AIDS cases. AIDS patients often have a history of multiple exposures to antibiotics for the treatment of sexually transmitted diseases acquired before AIDS becomes manifest. These antibiotics, themselves noxious influences, represent stresses that undermine the host's defensive reaction to the AIDS virus. As a consequence, the host's defenses retreat a "quantum jump", from the level where the virus's effects had been contained, to a deeper level. This defensive shift actually signifies that the host is more deeply disturbed than previously; the immune response has proven inadequate in coping with this intruder. If the host continues to be subjected to the effects of strong drugs, the disturbance will penetrate deeper and deeper levels; e.g. the central nervous system—the deepest level of involvement in AIDS virus infections.

The negative influence of drugs is not only quantitative but also qualitative, the former being the visible or direct side effects of drugs upon the human organism, and the latter being the subtle, long-range impact upon the natural defenses. The long-range impact is the destruction of the organism's inner ecology. After prolonged allopathic "therapies" a patient's defense system becomes confused and almost paralyzed, losing its capacity to initiate curative responses because such reactions are constantly counteracted by the intervention of some allopathic medicine.

On the other hand, most of the serious alternative therapies focus on strengthening the curative abilities of the organism. If the stimulus is curative or positive, a process of regeneration will begin and ultimately a real cure can take place. But the stimulus must be powerful and specific.

The confusion which exists today in the field of alternative methods of healing is due to the fact that the so-called practitioners of these therapeutic arts are not experts in their specialties and therefore cannot provide the individualized and absolutely specific treatment necessary for each case. The fault does not lie with the individuals who practice these therapies, but with the health authorities who have so far shown a frightening indifference in supporting alternative educational centers. There are a few exceptions in the U.S.A., such as schools of Osteopathy and Naturopathy. Individuals who want to learn an alternative therapeutic modality in depth usually cannot find an authoritative school or educational center. In desperation they turn to anybody who professes to teach these alternative therapies. Confusion and exploitation often result. For their part, medical authorities are contemptuous of alternative therapies; they promptly label them "quackery" and refuse to examine them further.

So convenient a response will not long remain tenable. The emergence of AIDS, CFIDS, candida and other new epidemics and diseases have already alarmed the unsuspecting public into questioning the assumptions of the allopathic bureaucracy.

15. During the process of changing levels through quantum jumps, the organism offers considerable resistance which can be transcended only by the intensity and quality of the stimuli (information).

At all times, the organism is automatically adjusting to the stresses received from the inner and outer environment. Thus in order to maintain a status quo or homeostasis, it puts up resistance in the form of minor and imperceptible changes within the body, which constantly reestablish the inner balance.

Yet there are positive and negative stimuli which, because of their quality and intensity, overthrow this resistance and initiate positive or negative processes.

If a friend of yours asks you to change your way of life, it is certain you will resist in the beginning; but if he keeps on giving you his reasons, and if these reasons strike a sensitive chord in you, you may opt for the change. It is the same with every kind of information. Initiating any real change will depend on how deep your need is for it, how much you appreciate it, and what kind of sensitivity—predisposition—you have towards it.

If you keep on hammering an organism with antibiotics, eventually, because of the strength of the stimulus, the organism will have to change its level of resistance and go to an even deeper level. Here we may cite the example of *Proteus*, a non-pathogenic organism (a natural inhabitant in the intestinal flora) which mutates to a pathogenic organism under continuous treatment with antibiotics given for milder infections. The overall health condition of the individual is thus degraded.

16. **A relatively healthy organism is at all times in a state of "sensitive balance" with a certain degree of "unpredictability" concerning the future. Any changes that may ensue because of a stimulus will depend on the organism's health—on all three planes—as well as the quality and intensity of the information (stimulus-stress) it receives.**

Because of its very nature, a healthy organism is in dynamic balance, which it tries to maintain at all cost. When the human organism has attained this balance and is in the best possible health, it exhibits a kind of vulnerability because of its dynamic, fluidic state. It seems that everything in its environment has to work for it now, harmoniously and conclusively, if it is to maintain this optimum, balanced condition. The tendency is to easily lose such an equilibrium under a strong negative or positive influence. Moving negatively is akin to "entropy"; moving positively is akin to evolution toward a higher level of existence.

It appears it is not so difficult for a negative stimulus to break down the first defenses of a healthily balanced organism, but once disturbed the organism will put up another line of defense that is much more difficult to break down. This means the stimulus necessary to push the disorder into deeper levels has to be much stronger and more invasive.

For example, let us look at the case of a chronic hay fever sufferer.

In the early years of this individual's life, it appeared that his hay fever condition began from "out of the blue" and without much provocation. In order for hay fever to be "suppressed" into an asthmatic condition, a very strong stressor or a very weak organism is needed. Such a state can come about from frequent use of antihistamines to relieve the hay fever. The mucous membranes of the nostrils become dry (the catarrh stops), and their responsiveness is destroyed by this treatment. But since the organism needs the relief afforded by a catarrh, it is now forced to mobilize its defenses on a deeper level in the bronchi in the form of an asthmatic condition.

Very seldom is this done automatically as a natural process. It is only when the organism is already too weak to keep the disturbance on a peripheral level (nostrils) that such a process develops automatically. But suppression is considerably easier to accomplish with chemical drugs such as antihistamines. The reason is that natural diseases have limited power over the organism; an inherent predisposition must exist before a natural disease invades deeper levels. But chemical drugs have an unlimited power over any organism when they are introduced into it in great quantities and for a sufficient length of time. If such a process is repeated over and over again, even the strongest organisms will succumb and allow the manifestation of new diseases.

The hypothesis in this treatise is that the HIV (Human Immunosuppressive Virus) would not have appeared and affected the human race in such an epidemic manner unless it had been preceded by widespread and frequent use of antibiotics which prepared the ground by breaking down the organism's immune system.

The people who became its first victims were almost exclusively those who had used huge quantities of such antibiotics. These drugs obviously broke down several lines of defense in the organism's immune system, rendering it susceptible to the virus. In the last chapter of this book I will expound on the logic of this hypothesis.

An organism can fall vulnerable to any kind of disease to which it is predisposed as long as there is a strong stress applied to it on a constant basis. It will soon be verified in research laboratories beyond any reasonable doubt that a predisposition is necessary before an individual can be affected by the HIV virus.

REFERENCES:

1. Principal toxic, allergic and other adverse effects of antimicrobial drugs. *Med Let 1968; 10: 73-76*

2. SANDERS DY: Rash associated with ampicillin in infectious mononucleosis. *Clin Pediat 1969; 8: 47-48*

3. SMITH JW, JOHNSON JE III, CLUFF LE: Studies on the epidemiology of adverse drug reactions: II. An evaluation of penicillin allergy. *N Engl J Med 1966; 274: 998-1002*

4. STEWART GT: Allergenic residues to penicillins. *Lancet 1967; 1: 1177-1183*

5. HAUSER WE, REMINGTON JS: Effect of antibiotics on the immune response. *Amer J Med 1982; 72: 711-716*

6. WING EG, REMINGTON JS: Delayed hypersensitivity and macrophage functions. In FUDENBERG HH, STITES DP,CALDWELL JL, WELLS JV, eds. *Basic and Clinical Immunology,* 3rd ed., Los Altos, California: Lange Medical Publications, 1980; 129-143

7. MUKERJEE P, SCHULDT S, KASIK JE: Effect of rifampin on cutaneous hypersensitivity to purified protein derivative in humans. *Antimicrob Agents Chemother 1973; 4: 607-611*

8. SILVERMAN M, LEE PR: *Pills, Profits & Politics.* Berkeley: University of California Press, Berkeley 1974; 259

Chapter 10

SATURATION

17. Once "critical" information has been received, the organism responds to it *instantaneously* by changing and rearranging itself to digest or process it. From that moment onwards, the organism cannot be changed further by this information or stimulus. A point of *saturation* is reached automatically.

This law is valid for the natural development of disease. It states that once a virus, bacterium or other microbe has affected an organism, once it has actually triggered the disease processes, immediate changes occur on an energy level which inhibit the further harassment of the organism by the intruder. After these changes occur, it is no longer possible for the organism to be affected by the *external* stimuli because its own chemistry has already changed in order to protect itself. As soon as the organism reaches the point of saturation, defense processes (symptoms) start to manifest.

If the opposite were true and the intruder could continue to affect the susceptible organism, every patient would necessarily die from the constant inflow of the virus, bacterium, etc., which exists in his immediate environment.

It should be explained here that although the external environmental conditions cannot affect the organism any longer, what takes place inside the organism is another story. The microorganism which has entered the body and found conducive conditions has the tendency to survive by rapidly multiplying. This process is inimical to the organism, which also wants to survive. That is why the organism soon starts to fight the intruder by putting up its first line of defense, manifesting a variety of signs and symptoms.

The host's defenses are immediately mobilized because it quickly recognizes the danger from contact with the pathological agent. As a consequence, its whole chemistry changes and the susceptibility ceases. The patient may now stay in the same environment in which he was initially infected but will probably recover and will not automatically be reinfected.

Chapter 11

THE NATURE OF THE CAUSE OF DISEASES

18. For disease to manifest, two prerequisite conditions must exist: the first is the sustaining cause of disease, the second is an exciting or triggering cause.

The first condition pertains to the predisposition of the organism and the second to the stressor or stimulus. Both these conditions must be present in order for certain symptomatology to manifest.

In this *Model* it is understood that the "exciting" causes of disease are not material but always dynamic (energy-like) in nature, whether they be bacteria, viruses, fungi or an influence such as grief.

It is true that disease is induced only as a consequence of a stress upon the organism. It has been increasingly evident that stressors are not only specific bacteria, viruses or pathological microorganisms, but also any type of mental or emotional upset (received from the environment) that creates a new situation with which the organism finds difficulty in coping. The bibliography on the subject of stress is vast and too long to be listed here, but I will mention that Hans Selye has focused a whole treatise upon the subject of stress called *The Stress of Life*.

As far as the organism is concerned, information or a specific pathological microorganism have similar capacities in initiating diseases. Therefore, when we talk about stimuli or stressors (stresses), we mean information that has significance for the organism and that is immediately recognized. Such stimuli we call the "exciting causes" of disease, whereas the inherent predisposition we call the "sustaining cause" of disease.

19. Information or stimuli can be received through:
a. The mental-spiritual plane
b. The emotional-psychic plane
c. The physical-instinctual plane

Different diseases may be triggered by stimuli received through the emotional or mental planes. This is something so well known today that few dispute or doubt it. Psychosomatic medicine deals exclusively with such conditions. All such conditions penetrate one's system through a process of feeling or thinking, while consequences can be felt on all levels: mental, emotional or physical, depending upon one's own predispositions.

This kind of stress is not "physical" in any way but is dynamic and energy-like. A similar dynamic, energy-like process takes place when the physical body gets sick from stressors that appear to be entirely material (microbes, bacteria, viruses etc.).

20. A disease will only manifest itself if the vibrational frequencies of the stimulus and the organism coincide.

A new energy state is instantly created, and this eventually changes the physicochemical inner environment such that the specific viruses, bacteria, etc., can thrive and multiply.

This idea is a bit advanced, but we will come back to it later in the book and elaborate. In the meantime, one has to ask the question: "How is it possible that the idea of an emotional or mental shock causing disease is acceptable, while that of the disease disturbance being energetic rather that just material is unacceptable?"

Another question that we might ask here: "Is it possible that after a stressor's encounter with an organism, conditions can develop within the system which might allow the mutation of innocuous microorganisms into ones which can cause pathology?"

Here is the opinion of Marc Lappé: "By making our own bodies the battlegrounds for chemical control of bacteria, we disrupt the natural ecological balance of the microorganisms that maintain the homeostasis of our internal and external surfaces... Overuse of antibiotics like penicillin may have participated in creating the soil for epidemics of antibiotic-resistant bacteria, and perhaps even AIDS."

These antibiotic-resistant organisms are not playthings. Many of them carry the same disease-causing properties as the germs that they replace. Moreover, they pose a long-term risk that has just not been projected yet, one that threatens the present "antibiotic-safe" generation of Americans. Infections of the 1980s were more difficult to treat and control than were their predecessors.

Chapter 12

UNIVERSAL ENERGY-CONSTRUCTION OF THE MODEL

The three planes of human existence cannot be separate or unconnected. There must be an essential underlying binding force.

21. All three levels of functioning are interconnected by a universal or cosmic energy field which is neutral in character and quality. The function of this energy is to animate everything in the Universe, including the triplex of body, mind and emotions of the human being. Each plane uses this basic energy and transforms it to suit its particular needs and functions. This type of energy is the *substratum* through which all physical manifestations can take place.

In a previous chapter we presented the concept of such a force and how it has been described by different scientists and metaphysicians. It has neutral qualities (neither good or bad) apart from those basic qualities inherent in a force. This very primal force attains different qualities according to the specific material manifestation that it animates.

It is that which gives "life" and enormous energy to every material thing. Einstein's formula and nuclear fission have shown us the actual amount of energy encapsulated in matter. It was his conception that everything existing in our material world is nothing but energy fields.

In spite of similar statements from recognized and celebrated scientists, established medicine insists on treating the human body as a machine or chemical factory, totally ignoring its real nature and structure and the natural laws that support it.

Today the presence of such an energy structure is becoming more and more apparent. This concept creates a need which must be dealt with by scientists, researchers and health practitioners.[3-24]

Universal or cosmic energy is an unlimited depot which man will soon consciously tap. The scientists working in physics with "small clusters" deal closely with this idea. We can draw pure, unlimited energy from this depot and apply it in a million ways.

Established medicine has concentrated its research and efforts in the past decades on only the physicochemical part of the human being. To continue in the same manner is somewhat of a "blind act" since it ignores the existing realities and needs of the human organism.

As I wrote in the foreword, my main purpose in producing this small treatise was to point out the fallacies of modern therapeutics while presenting a new hypothesis with renewed hope for this important branch of science. In this short work I cannot possibly give all the pertinent examples and explanations for everyone to fully understand my viewpoint; but I hope to give enough evidence that more dedicated scientists will start looking in the right direction. I shall be content if this initial exposure to the *Model* initiates some fruitful discussions.

22. The organism is constructed in such a manner that the more important, sensitive and precious organs are the most protected in order to ensure the safety and continuing existence of the organism. An optimum construction delineating both the idea of hierarchy and that of protection can be depicted symbolically by a truncated cone format.

In *Figure 20,* a diagrammatic model symbolically shows that the physical body envelops and contains the emotional and mental spheres. The diagram also represents the different lines of defense that potentially exist in the body. There are correspondences between the physical organs and the emotional and mental functions.

The three energy planes of the organism are represented symbolically by three truncated cones, each one overlapping the other with the physical plane on the periphery and the mental plane in the center. What this means is that the physical-material plane, which is the grossest and least vulnerable, comes in direct contact with the physical environment, while the other two parts, being of greater importance and sensitivity, need more protection and thus lie deeper within. This is especially true of the mental-spiritual plane, which is in the very center.

The vertical lines of the cones, if projected, would meet at one point, thereby symbolizing the solitary and unique character of the individual.

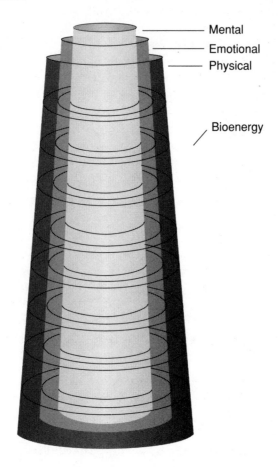

Figure 20: A symbolic model of the physical, emotional and mental spheres.

23. The three cones should be understood primarily as separate areas constructed out of many complex levels of organizational patterns or energy fields. Each of the main planes can be identified by its own vibrational frequency.

These vibrational frequencies are:

Mental Energy (M_e) :   fast frequency
Emotional Energy (E_e) :   medium frequency
Physical Energy (P_e) :   low frequency

The fields are very intense and dense in the material-physical plane, less so on the emotional plane, and even less on the mental plane. The energy used by all these planes comes from the general source of **universal energy**.

It appears that each individual, from the moment of birth, is endowed with a certain amount of "seed" energy that determines his lifespan (outside of any unpredictable circumstances). Theoretically, the length of time (lifespan) is determined by this energy plus one's genetic predisposition.

I believe that in the not-too-distant future we will be able to predict the degree of health of an individual and his probable lifespan. Measurements may be taken at certain years of his life that will give precise indications as to his possible strengths and weaknesses. There will be tests to measure physical strength and emotional soundness or resilience, and even more sophisticated tests will measure mental abilities and strengths. It is not in the scope of this book to discuss the various detailed tests that could determine the overall degree of health of a given individual at a particular time; I wish only to point out the numerous possibilities awaiting us in the future. Once one had such test results, preventive measures could be taken not only to protect but also to enhance health.

REFERENCES:

1. LAPPÉ M: *When Antibiotics Fail*. Berkeley, California: North Atlantic Books, 1986
2. CAPRA F: *The Tao of Physics*. Berkeley, California: Shambhala Publications, Inc., 1975
3. ADAMENKO VG: Electrodynamics of living systems. *J Paraphysics* 1970; 4: 113-120
4. ALEXANDER HS: Biomagnetics—the biological effects of magnetic fields. *Amer J Med Electronics* 1962; 1(4): 181-187
5. BARNARD RD: *Biologic Systems' Magnetic Susceptibility*. Biomedical Sciences Instrumentation 1963: Vol. 1. New York: Plenum Press, 143-156

6. BARTHONY M: *Biological Effects of Magnetic Fields.* Vol. 2. New York: Plenum Press, 1971

7. BEAL JB: Electrostatic Fields, Electromagnetic Field, and Ions: Mind/Body/Environment Interrelationships. *Sixth Annual Meeting of the Neuroelectric Soc, Vol 6, Snowmass-at-Aspen, Colorado*

8. BECKER RO: Relationship of the Geomagnetic Environment to Human Biology. *New York J Med 1963; 63: 2215-2219*

9. BOHM D: *Quantum Theory.* New York: Prentice-Hall, 1951

10. BOHM D: *Wholeness and the Implicate Order.* London: Routledge & Kegan Paul

11 BOHM D, HILEY B: On the Intuitive Understanding of Nonlocality as Implied by Quantum Theory. *Foundations of Physics, 1975; Vol 5: 93-109*

12. CLYNES M: Biocybernetics of the dynamic communication of emotions and qualities. *Science 1970; 170: 764-765*

13. COHEN D: Magnetic Fields of the Human Body. *Physics Today 1975; August, 34-43*

14. EDDINGTON AS: *New Pathways in Science.* Cambridge, England: Cambridge University Press, 1935

15. EDDINGTON AS: *The Philosophy of Physical Science.* Cambridge, England: Cambridge University Press, 1939

16. HEISENBERG W: *Physics and Beyond.* New York: Harper & Row

17. KHODOLOV YA: *The Effect of Electromagnetic and Magnetic Fields on the Central Nervous System.* Moscow: Nauka, 1966

18. KRIPPNER S, RUBIN D: *The Energies of Consciousness.* New York: Interfac Book, Gordon and Breach, 1975, 130

19. MUTSCHALL V: Biological Effects of Magnetic Fields. *Foreign Science Bull 1969; 5(2): 13-36*

20. PRESMAN AS: *Electromagnetic Fields and Life.* New York: Plenum Press, 1970

21. RUSSO F, CALDWELL WE: Biomagnetic Phenomena: Some Implications for the Behavioral and Neurophysiological Sciences. *Genetic Psychol Monographs 1971; 84: 177-243*

22. SZENT-GYORGI A: *Introduction to a Submolecular Biology.* New York; Academic Press, 1960

23. SMIRNOV BM: *Introduction to Plasma Physics.* Moscow: Mir Publishers, 1977

24. WHITEHEAD AN: *Science and the Modern World.* New York: Macmillan, 1926

Chapter 13

THE SIGNIFICANCE OF THE PLANES

In the near future the significance of the mental and emotional planes will be more widely appreciated, and people will realize their importance to overall well-being. Our educational systems will be reorganized with this in mind, and education will really become a more human endeavor. Students will be happy to go to such educational centers where the wonders of science and art will be taught to them.

I envision schools where Beethoven's symphonies and Rembrandt's paintings will take up equal teaching time with physics and chemistry; and where the philosophical teachings of ancient Greece will be taught along with Egyptian, Hebrew and Indian mystical philosophies.

Education, as it stands today, is unbalanced. It fails because it is based on developing human intelligence and physical strength to the exclusion of the development of the emotional and spiritual part of the human being. It is also based on competition and ambition instead of the love and wisdom inherent in us all.

At the moment, technology has overwhelmed the individual and crushed him under its spell. Human beings of all intellects become slaves of this technology. It is progressing so fast that the individual has to work more and more in order to catch up with the "opportunities" it offers. Nobody sits back to contemplate; even during our holidays we run here and there, winding down only when it is time to return home and to continue our crazy race for material gains.

In the West we have finally managed to amass tremendous material gains, but we have paid for them with unbelievable spiritual loss. The price we will pay will also be great in terms of our health.[1]

24. As the *Model* is constructed, it can easily be recognized that a correspondence of ideas exists among the mental, emotional and physical planes. Certain emotional traits correspond to certain organs and functions of the physical body or mind and vice-versa.

It might be too early or too presumptuous to speak about a correspondence between the way we feel or think and the condition of our physical organs. But from my experience in treating people, and from the experience of many well-trained physicians, it appears that the idea is valid.[2-8] People with a certain fear will develop a corresponding disturbance in one of their physical organs.[9] Rigidity of character may result in rigidity of the muscular structure, especially the tendons.[10] A person who is very tight with his money may develop constipation, or someone who has undertaken too much responsibility may develop stiffness in his neck area. One who is prone to depression may develop problems with his liver, and one whose mind is too hesitant about vital issues may develop some kind of paralysis. These are only general examples suggesting a direction for future research, and are neither precise nor conclusive. There are so many parameters to be considered in such research that in this book I only want to introduce the idea.

REFERENCES:

1. MUMFORD L: *The Pentagon of Power.* Vol. 2, The Myth of Megamachine. New York: Harcourt Brace, 1970
2. ALEXANDER F: *Psychosomatic Medicine.* New York: Norton, 1950
3. DORFMAN W: *Closing the Gap Between Medicine and Psychiatry.* Proceedings of the First International Congress of the Academy of Psychosomatic Medicine, E DUNLOP, ed. New York: Excerpta Medica Foundation, 1967: 11-14
4. ENGEL GL: The psychosomatic approach to individual susceptibility to disease. *Gastroenterology, 1974, 67: 1085-1093*
5. FRIEDIMAN SB, GLASCOC LA: Psychologic factors and resistance to infectious disease. *Ped Clin N Amer 1966; 13: 315-335*
6. LACEY GI: Differential emphasis in somatic response to stress. *Psychosomatic Medicine, 1952; 14, 71*
7. LIPOWSKI ZJ: Psychosomatic Medicine in the seventies: An overview (102 references). *Amer J Psychiat 1977; 134(3), 233-244*

8. PELLETIER KR: *A Perspective Approach to Psychosomatic Medicine.* BRESSLER D, GORDON J, JAFFE D, eds. Body, mind and health: Toward an integral medicine. Washington, DC: National Institute of Mental Health, 1979

9. WORCESTER J: *Psychological Correspondences.* Boston: Massachusetts New Church Union, 1931

10. REICH W: *Selected Writings.* New York: Farrar, Straus & Giroux, 1979

Chapter 14

PREDISPOSITIONS

25. The body is born with certain weaknesses or areas that are potentially responsible for triggering disease. Such weaknesses will be called predispositions.

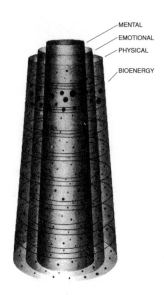

MENTAL
EMOTIONAL
PHYSICAL
BIOENERGY

Figure 21: Latent predisposition of the organism.

Predispositions are formed in the following manner and circumstances:

    a. Hereditary complexes (genetic codes) from the parents as well as their ancestors

    b. Inappropriate treatments received during one's lifetime

    c. External circumstances that force the individual to think in a specific way or to develop certain negative feelings

a. Hereditary complexes (genetic codes) from the parents as well as their ancestors.

Many hereditary predispositions are well known today through genetic research. It is already possible, through sophisticated laboratory examinations, to determine the diseases to which a particular individual is predisposed.

Established medicine has made great strides in this field. Various geneticists have come to the conclusion that certain genetic predispositions are factors in the manifestation of certain diseases. Of course, it is easier for established medicine to accept such a role of predispositions in the manifestation of chronic rather than acute disease. Inherent predisposition is exhibited under the stress of certain negative environmental factors in such diseases as diabetes, hypertension and coronary heart disease. A new term labeled "personal immunity" is introduced in the field of acute infectious disease by allopathic medicine in order to explain the "unreasonable" and "unexplained" fact that although many people may be infected by the same agent, they do not all manifest the expected disease. On the other hand "personal sensitivity" is used to explain the opposite phenomenon, namely the existence of hypersensitivity towards certain pathological agents.[1-4]

Alternative medicine and especially Homeopathy[5] have long maintained that a predisposition is necessary for the manifestation of a disease.

Even today, established medicine makes no use of the concept of predisposition either therapeutically or in its research. As a result, drugs are prescribed to sensitive patients with devastating results.

The effects of primaquine, phenacetin, sulfonamides, furadantin and aspirin upon persons with a lack of G-6-PD enzyme are already well known. Unfortunately, there are also other drugs whose inappropriate use has led to the discovery of different genetic anomalies and consequently, predispositions. Such drugs include: isoniazid, succinyl choline, H_2O_2, anesthetic drugs, and anticoagulants.[4]

Perhaps the only cases dealing with such "sensitivities" that established medicine has taken into consideration are the tests given to patients for penicillin sensitization.

b. Inappropriate treatments received during one's lifetime.

Today, inappropriate treatment is responsible for many diseases. Allergic conditions are at an all-time high because of the inordinate use of drugs that deeply affect the immune system. The excessive use of drugs is responsible for the development of a multitude of new pathological conditions. Of course, the most classic example remains the sensitivity towards penicillin that has developed because of the wide use of this drug.

The (already high) [6-16] statistics revealing the number of iatrogenic diseases take into consideration only those patients who appear to fall ill **directly** after their exposure to allopathic drugs. But there are many more cases that suffer from the long-term effects of allopathic drugs; these cases are not included in the statistics because the beginning of illness does not coincide with the time of treatment. There are pharmacologists who support this contention and classify the side effects of allopathic drugs as short-term and long-term, the latter being the more dangerous because they are unpredictable and have a widespread influence on humanity (e.g. carcinogenesis).[5]

A person will naturally ask the question, "If there are so many documented cases of harmful side effects from drugs, is it possible that all other patients who received the same drugs in the same quantity have escaped the consequences completely?"

Paradoxical as it may seem, research scientists who work for pharmaceutical companies never ask such questions.

The truth of the matter is that every patient, according to his specific sensitivities and predispositions, incurs a relative side effect that takes one of the following forms:

1. Those patients who are very sensitive to a drug and at the same time are in a very precarious state of health may suffer a fatal outcome from the treatment.
2. Those who are sensitive to the drug but whose health is better will have severe side effects but will survive.
3. Those who are not very sensitive to the drug but whose health is poor will develop long-term effects after the treatment; the organism will fall subtly and insidiously into a second line of defense because of the treatment.

4. Those who are not sensitive to the drug and whose overall state of health is quite good will survive the treatment and will manifest only mild, temporary side effects which will go away without further disturbance.

Of course, there are other subgroups within these classifications, but here it will suffice to specify only those mentioned above. The gist of the matter is that after an enormous assault on the organism by massive doses of allopathic drugs, there are varied side effects exhibited by different individuals that defy classification; therefore, the real extent of the harm done by allopathic drugs will never be known. Such "drugging" can create new predispositions and convert existing ones into full-blown diseases.

I regret having to be so emphatic about drug side effects because I do recognize the value of allopathic drugs in certain situations. My principal objection is with the manner in which these drugs have been utilized by the established medical system. From my perspective these drugs have on the whole been more harmful than beneficial.[15]

c. *External circumstances that force the individual to think in a specific way or to develop certain negative feelings.*

Negative thoughts and feelings resulting from some unfortunate event in life are the third way of creating predispositions to disease. We will take as an example the case of parents who have an invalid child. For some, this event is taken in the right way; it is accepted and faced in a calm manner. For others, this same event becomes a source of constant grief and upset and daily torture. These constant negative feelings or thoughts will eventually predispose the organism to some serious health problem even though the person initially appears quite healthy. The same thing happens with any kind of grief that remains as a source of emotional or mental suffering for a long time.

26. Predisposition is "a potential condition" which may or may not manifest as a pathological state during the lifespan of an individual. Its manifestation will

depend on the quality of the individual's life and the number and intensity of the stresses.

This is something that needs little explanation as it is rather self-evident; namely, a person may be born with an undermined constitution, predisposed to different diseases, yet may not get sick if he lives a healthy life and is lucky enough not to encounter hostile stimuli that will trigger his predispositions.

One can find such individuals in remote places where the "chemicals" of contemporary life have not yet overwhelmed the area and where life has a different rhythm than in our modern cities.

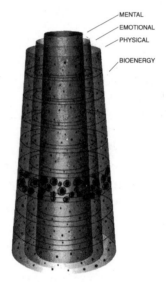

Figure 22: Activated predisposition.

What is important to understand is that many chronic diseases manifested in people living in contemporary societies are becoming more and more common. This is due to increased ingestion of prescription and non-prescription drugs, environmental pollution and inadequate diet. All of these factors trigger existing predispositions on the one hand, and on the other, prepare the way for creating new ones.

Similarly, there are people born with excellent hereditary traits from the healthiest of parents who may still die quite young, due to the fact that in their case two out of three of the factors that we have discussed are extremely negative. These negative factors are inappropriate medical treatment coupled with very difficult external circumstances, which together generate a persistently negative emotional state.

It is also possible for a person born with certain predispositions to disease to rise above them by obtaining correct treatment and living "properly." It is quite conceivable that a person born with the predisposition to die at the age of 75 years may live up to age 85 or even 100 if he follows a "right way of living."

We actually lengthen or shorten our potential lifespan by the way we treat ourselves and the way we live our lives. The much-publicized notions of an extended lifespan for western people are definitely misleading. Before the appearance of AIDS, the following was written in 1976 in *DHSS Prevention and Health, Everybody's Business*: "Every year health expenditure rises without any increase in the benefits to the population. In the last thirty years life expectancy has not risen for anybody over the age of 45 at all."

Illich, using as reference the paper of Charles Stewart, *Allocation of Resources to Health*,[17] states, "In contrast to environmental improvements and modern non-professional health measures, the specific medical treatment of people is never significantly related to a decline in the compound disease burden or to a rise in life expectancy... It is therefore ironic that during this unique boom in health care the United States has established another 'first'. Shortly after the boom started, the life expectancy for adult American males began to decline and is now expected to decline even further." [15]

The quality of life has also dropped dramatically. In many instances, modern civilized man is already "dead" at the age of 35. He is "dead" because the quality of his health has deteriorated. There are mental and emotional disturbances which began at an early age and continue for a very long time; there is no joy or happiness in life, but only a wretched existence that drags along, artificially supported by drugs. Today people may live up to 60 or 70 years, but with osteoarthritis, rheumatoid arthritis, allergies, asthma, heart conditions, neuromuscular disorders, epilepsy, diabetes, mental diseases, Alzheimer's disease, idiocy, cancer or AIDS. What kind of life are they leading and at what cost and suffering to themselves, their families and their societies?

Has anybody calculated the total number of people "dragging along" in our western societies with very serious chronic conditions, and the total cost paid by different governments to prolong their ordeal? Can established medicine pride itself on such attainments?

Why is it that the total cost of health care has reached such unprecedented heights in these countries? Such costs could only be justified if everyone in these societies were sick or disabled for a considerable length of time. Yet often established medicine quotes statistics that are not representative of the real picture, and we naively believe their claims. Very few individuals have ever pointed the finger at established medicine and blamed it for the state of health in which we find ourselves today.

27. Every organism has different levels of predispositions that under stress can be triggered in stages.

The first group of predispositions to be triggered in the life of a person will be the least serious medically. If the organism continues to receive harmful stimulation, especially from chemical drugs, then the second line of resistance comes into action and a new level of predisposition is activated. In such an instance the disturbance automatically goes deeper and becomes more serious. The person actually dies when his main level of predisposition (his weakest point) has been activated.

This is what has happened with AIDS. Constant venereal infections in conjunction with repeated assaults from chemical drugs have broken down the defenses of young and initially healthy individuals and brought them to the last stage of their defenses.

If the hypothesis advanced in this *Model* is correct, one can easily understand the confusion that would be created within the organism if antibiotics continued to be prescribed for pneumocystis carinii pneumonia (one of the end stages of AIDS).

28. There are different degrees of attraction between the organism and various pathological agents. The severity of the disease is directly proportional to the degree of attraction.

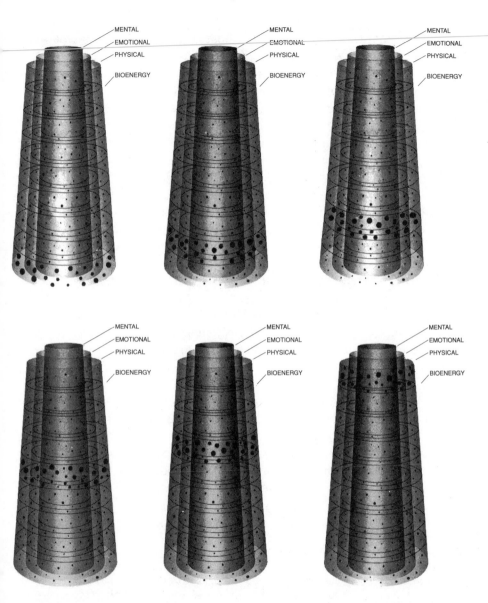

Figure 23: Different levels on which the main predisposition of different organisms may lie.

When the predisposition is activated by a stimulus toward which the organism maintains a great degree of susceptibility, we witness the manifestation of sudden, serious signs and symptoms.

The attraction between the host and stimulus must be of great magnitude in order for the above to happen. This mutual attraction and the ensuing results take place instantaneously because this recognition occurs on an energy level. The initial embrace of the stimulus with the organism is the primary event; the symptoms come later. These symptoms are the child that is born after the "embrace" and resulting "fertilization," and after the "incubation period" in which the disease has been conceived but has not yet manifested itself.

The greater the attraction between the host and stimulus, the stronger the child (disease). As the attraction or susceptibility lessens, so does the severity of the manifested symptoms.

This principle explains why some people will develop quite dramatic symptomatology and die soon after an infection while others, given the same circumstances, will recover with considerable ease.

Yet in spite of different predispositions, different reactions to pathological agents and different general states of health, allopathic physicians still prescribe the same drugs to people with a specific disease, ignoring the peculiar sensitivities and particular idiosyncracies of these individuals.

People are under the impression that they will die unless they take certain antibiotics or whatever medicine is prescribed. This is a delusion not even supported by the medical community itself. There is much research available today to show that different treatments given during epidemics have had very little or nothing to do with the decline of the epidemic.[18-20]

"However, when antibiotics are prescribed without adequate testing to determine the vulnerabilities of the infecting organism, or when the infection has already gone on a long time, problems are the rule and not the exception. As we have seen, one of these problems is the emergence of new strains of bacteria that are resistant to the particular antibiotic being used. ...The previous error of using penicillin to treat every respiratory illness even suspected of being bacterial was repeated with staph infections. Even those infections that would have responded to conservative treatment—such as lancing and draining boils—were systematically treated without any clear effort to establish patients' need or the susceptibility of the bacteria in question." [11]

REFERENCES:

1. EMERY AEH: *Heredity, Disease and Man. Genetics in Medicine.*
   Berkeley: University of California Press, 1968
2. LINKS JL: *Extrachromosomal Inheritance.* Prentice-Hall, 1964
3. STEINBERG AG, BEARN AG: *Progress in Medical Genetics.* (Vol.
   VIII) W. Heinemann Med. Books, 1972
4. EMERY AEH: *Elements of Medical Genetics.* Livingstone, 1968
5. WINTROBE: *The Therapeutic Millenium and its Price. Drugs in our
   Society.* Baltimore: The Johns Hopkins Press.
6. SIMMONS HE: An overview of public policy and infectious diseases.
   Ann Inter Med 1978; 89 (Part 2): 821-825
7. FINLAND M: And the walls come tumbling down: more antibiotic
   resistance, and now the pneumonococcus. *N Engl J Med 1978; 299:
   770-771*
8. FINLAND M: Changing patterns of common bacterial pathogens to
   antimicrobial agents. *Ann Inter Med 1972; 76: 1009-1013*
9. FINLAND M: Superinfections in the antibiotic era. *Postgraduate Med
   1973; 54: 175-183*
10. FINLAND M: Emergence of antibiotic resistance in hospitals, 1935-
    1975. *Rev Infect Dis 1980; 1: 4-21*
11. KUNIN CM: Antibiotic accountability. *N Engl J Med 1979; 301:
    380-381*
12. KUNIN CM, et al: Use of antibiotics: A brief exposition of the problem
    and some tentative solutions. *Ann Inter Med 1973; 79: 555-561*
13. KUNIN CM: Problems of antibiotic usage: Definitions, causes and
    proposed solutions. *Ann Inter Med 1978; 89(Part 2): 802-805*
14. DIXON RE: Nosocomial infections: a continuing problem. *Postgraduate
    Med 1977; 62: 95-109*
15. ILLICH I: *Limits to Medicine. Medical Nemesis: The Expropriation of
    Health.* Pelican Books, 1977
16. FOUCAULT M: *The Birth of the Clinic.* Translated by A. M. Sheridan
    Smith. New York: Pantheon, 1973
17. STEWART CT: Allocation of resources to health. *J Human Resources
    6, 1971; no.1, 3-121*
18. McKEOWN T: *The Role of Medicine. Dream, Mirage or Nemesis?*
    Oxford: Basil Blackwell, 1979
19. McKINLAY JB, McKINLAY SM: The questionable contribution of
    medicine to the decline of mortality in the United States in the
    twentieth century. *Milbank Mem Fund Q, 1977; 55: 405-428*
20. PORTER RR: The contribution of the biological and medical sciences to
    human welfare. *Presidential address to the British Association for the
    Advancement of Science, Swansea Meeting, 1971*
21. LAPPÉ M: *When Antibiotics Fail. Restoring the Ecology of the Body.*
    Berkeley, California: North Atlantic Books, 1986

Chapter 15

THE DEFENSE SYSTEM

29. The human organism possesses a very complex defense mechanism that helps it maintain its optimum balance. This mechanism transcends its physical components and operates on an energy level.

Some components already known on the physical level are:

a. Immune system
b. Reticuloendothelial system
c. Sympathetic-parasympathetic system
d. Hormonal system
e. Lymphatic system

The organism mobilizes one or more components of the defense system depending on the particular stressor and its singular susceptibility to it. But the whole of the defense mechanism is too complex to be known in its entirety.

What is important to understand is that when the immune system acts or reacts, it is responding to an order given from a "central intelligence source" which is within and at the same time above these systems. The order of mobilization of a system and how this is coordinated is something beyond the capacity of even the greatest artificial intelligence known today. This superintelligence which exists in the organism should be envisioned as an energy-field structure, a supercomputer situated at a level that cannot be thought of in purely material terms (as in chemistry, in purely physicochemical terms).[1]

30. When a stressor exercises a strong influence (due to the susceptibility of the organism to it), then the threshold of "hesitant balance" is crossed and the organism moves via a "quantum jump" to a new pattern of minor coherence (more confusion). It seems that for every given state of health there are

several probabilities to which the organism may jump, via a quantum leap, when it is under pressure from a "critical" stimulus.

Let us now define our terms. "Hesitant balance" describes that delicate balance between degrees of health and disease. We can visualize this balance as a man walking on a tightrope. He is fine as long as he has a footing on the tightrope; but once he slips, he falls to one side or the other or to another level, and the "balance of health" is disturbed.

It is known that electronic orbits are perceived as energy bands or standing-waves in accordance with quantum theory. We know that electrons are induced to change orbits by one of two factors:

a. External excitation (energy gain or loss)
b. Nuclear disturbances

"The apparent disappearance and reappearance of the electron between orbits is due to the fact that the planetary electron has no identity unless along a nuclear standing-wave (i.e., energy band)."[2]

The external excitation is the "exciting cause" or stressor in illness, while "nuclear disturbance" is the maintaining cause or the inherent predisposition.

As regards "nuclear disturbances," we have to understand more specifically the internal changes within the organism that allow for the development of a disease.

A stressor (a pathological agent) can be thought of as the "electron" which determines health or disease. It has no "identity" or power by itself. It is a non-existent entity as far as the organism is concerned, but it attains its power once there is an attraction between it and the organism and a bond established between them. In other words, its power is derived and manifested from the organism's special susceptibility to it. A stressor may be quite virulent and yet not have the capacity to effect any changes within a specific organism because that organism is not susceptible to it. An example of this is that carriers of the HIV-AIDS virus may not exhibit any symptoms of the disease.

It is only when the internal conditions of the organism are conducive to the development of a specific pathological agent that a disease process begins. The virus or bacteria can be within the organism and yet produce no disease (hepatitis B, etc.).[3] For instance, why is it that when you overexert yourself a common cold or influenza may develop? In order to provide the virus with the opportunity to thrive, one has to stress the organism to produce the appropriate chemical changes.

Such ideas are common and almost universally accepted today, yet they have not been applied to research or therapeutics and are either ignored or misinterpreted.

Everybody is trying to find out where the AIDS virus has come from, and nobody seems to realize that it might have been with us all along, the only difference being that now the conditions are ripe for infection within millions of organisms.

Today we see the disease in its epidemic form simply because a great number of organisms have been undermined through venereal diseases, drugs and general pollution, so that their immune systems have become incapable of combating the virus.

From the knowledge we have today on the mutation of microorganisms under stress (chemical changes within the body), we may deduce that the virus could have sprung from **an endogenous process** of constant mutations of different microorganisms.

In the early stages of the AIDS epidemic, there was already a great number of humans who automatically manifested the virus through a series of mutations because of a great predisposition towards this virus. These human organisms then became the potential sources of infection for other humans who were similarly prepared to accept the virus.

The live organism is in a dynamic state which accepts change, be it large or small. It is in a state where an electron can move between orbits and therefore disappear or reappear, determining whether the organism will be thrown off balance or will remain in balance. For example, how many times during the day does your mood change? When you are in a bad, depressed or anxious mood, there are deep changes within your system that fluctuate according to your external and internal conditions. It is obvious that your mood not only changes temporarily but also for longer periods of time and may, depending on the stress, change permanently. In the case of chronic depression we may say that the electron which formerly maintained the balance is

gone for good and consequently, the organism has jumped to a
different reality in relation to its energy state.

When something of this nature occurs in the organism, then
we can conclude that it has suddenly changed levels in a manner
which can be understood only as an energy change or a quantum
jump.

The organism always seems to hesitate as to which way it
should go. Depending on several parameters, there is a choice of
different probabilities which the organism may follow given
different stresses (theory of uncertainty).[5]

Perhaps such a state is more easily understood when we
examine the cases where weather changes trigger a better or
worse state of health. We can all accept that electrical potentials
of the atmosphere affect human organisms, and there are many
individual cases which suffer intensely from these barometric
changes.

31. Diseases are nothing but the activation and consequent manifestation of the existing predispositions in response to stress.

So far we have arrived logically at the conclusion that for
diseases to manifest, they must have an underlying, continuing
cause which is **not** the bacteria, virus or fungus, but the deep-
seated predisposition of the organism. Bacteria or viruses will
appear as soon as the internal conditions of the organism
change; in this manner the organism becomes an ideal breeding
ground for them.

Even if the appropriate bacteria or virus is not present, they
can still manifest (in the organism) through a series of mutations from similar preexisting microorganisms.

If this hypothesis is true, the whole concept and cornerstone
belief of classical medicine—that bacteria, viruses, fungi, etc.,
are the causes of disease—will collapse.

This assumption has great repercussions therapeutically and
also for research because there is an enormous difference between "killing" the invading organisms—something that
allopathic medicine tries to do—and maintaining the defense
system in the best possible condition, as suggested by the *Model*.

This cornerstone idea of "killing the invader" put forth by
established medicine has been so entrenched in our way of

thinking that changing it borders on the heretical. Yet unless we decide to really look at the facts with an open mind and a sincere desire to understand what is going on, we will never solve the riddle of these vicious epidemics. Today, the worst of these epidemics is called AIDS; tomorrow some other name may take precedence.

I do believe that if we carry on in the same way and continue using such large quantities of strong chemicals, new epidemics worse than AIDS will soon appear.

32. The totality of the organism's response under stress creates a pattern of symptomatology that is uniquely individual for that patient. According to this principle, there cannot be a generalized treatment for a specific type of disorder.

Specific stressors like bacteria, microbes, viruses, etc., bring about gross reactions (disease symptoms) that on a superficial level look quite similar in everyone. Yet looking closer at each person's symptomatology we perceive individualized reactions in different organisms that signify the **individual** response to stress. If the same treatment is given to everyone it will probably be to the detriment of the organism, which will have to face not only the disease but also the chemicals used to counteract the disease.

In established medicine, there may be talk about the need for a holistic approach in treating patients, but in actual practice the exact opposite occurs—the same medicine is prescribed for every patient with a specific disease.

In England, physicians established the Holistic British Medical Association to persuade people about their sincerity and beliefs in these principles.

It seems that orthodox medical people realize that the precepts of alternative medicine are correct. They acknowledge that treatment should address the whole individual in his mental, emotional and physical totality rather than only his local, physical manifestations. When it comes to actual practice, however, they frequently have no other option but to give the official treatment specific for a disease. The conventional type of treatment is supported and maintained by research groups and promoted by certain pharmaceutical companies with interests in mind.

The idea that the FDA (U.S. Food and Drug Administration) exerts some control over the distribution of products to the American market and works for the best interests of the public is, in my opinion, misleading, because the people in the administration are usually of the same mind as the researchers. They do not adhere to or apply different principles in viewing the efficacy and danger of the drugs. So, although their intervention prevents to some extent extremely dangerous drugs from flooding the market with devastating results, the FDA does not solve the whole problem.

Silverman and Lee quote various disastrous examples of pharmaceutical promotion, such as the sulfanilamide affair in 1938, the chloramphenicol affair in the 1950s, the MER/29 (triparanol) affair in 1959, the affair of oral contraceptives, and the case of oral anti-diabetic agents.[6]

"The welter of documents available in the offices of the SEC confirm the conclusion from interviews with industry executives: bribery is routine and widespread in the international pharmaceutical industry and large amounts of money are involved. Almost every type of person who can affect the interests of the industry has been the subject of bribes by pharmaceutical companies: doctors, hospital administrators, cabinet ministers, health inspectors, customs officers, tax assessors, drug registration officials, factory inspectors, pricing officials, and political parties.

"....The problem of suppression of facts is widespread. A typical case occurs along the following lines: a toxicological study has been conducted and gives an equivocal result or a result unfavorable to the product. A second study is conducted and at times even a third in which the dose levels are adjusted or the protocols modified in such a way that eventually a result favorable to the applicant's product is obtained. Only the result favorable to the applicant's product is submitted to the regulatory authority....Microscopic examinations of histopathological slides may be made by more than one pathologist each of whom may have come to different conclusions, yet only the conclusions favorable to the drug are submitted to the regulatory authority. On one occasion where such a situation has been detected the applicant with a dismissive gesture said 'that investigator gives the wrong results; we will not use him again.' (This attitude reveals the commercial pressure that can be brought to bear on an investigator by the threat of loss of future work.)"[7]

33. **Signs and symptoms are not the disease per se, but an expression of the unique way in which the individual's defense system is trying to eradicate the disease.**

In effect this principle says that fever, edema, pain, chills, convulsions, anxiety, depression and, in general, any symptom that the organism may produce under stress is not the disease per se, but the means by which the organism is trying to get rid of the disease.

Karl Menninger in his book *The Vital Balance* takes up this point quite aptly and states:

"...These phenomena are symptoms in the sense that they indicate that something is wrong and that help is needed...At first this was rejected as utter nonsense; who on earth would wish to have a headache? Who would want to be paralyzed? Who would crave even the minor discomforts and disabilities?

"...our purpose in this book is to emphasize the economic interpretation, the function of the symptom in the maintenance of organismic equilibrium and integrity."

"...Mental illness is not an invasion but a defensive reaction."

"...Twenty years ago the late Robert Lindner put it brilliantly thus: 'It has been brought home to me ever more forcibly that the aggression, the hostility, the rejection of authority, the migratory tendencies, the impulsiveness, the destructive and blind lashing-out of the psychopath—all of these are homeostatic adjustments operating to restore a dynamic equilibrium within the personality.' "[8]

34. A symptom is therefore a useful and necessary condition that should be freely expressed rather than suppressed.

On this principle rests the greatest difference between allopathic and alternative medicine. Everyone who practices alternative medicine today, including the converts from medical colleges, understands and respects this principle. Scientists from all fields perceive its truth immediately, and I have never met a patient, educated or not, who has not understood this principle.

Established medicine's whole concept concerning diseases would have changed if only this principle had been understood and appreciated.

According to the allopathic way of thinking, it is logical that the symptoms which appear should be eliminated, since they constitute the disease and are dangerous to the organism's survival. But if only some symptoms are eliminated by such treatment, it may prove detrimental to the organism as a whole, because some of its important decisions to defend the whole would not only be ignored, but also suppressed. Such practice is certain to bring the immune system and its defenses to a state of deficiency and confusion.

"The function of the symptom" is "in the maintenance of organismic equilibrium and integrity. This, we feel, has been neglected and is only recently coming to be fully appreciated."[8]

When under unbearable stress, the organism will manifest signs and symptoms that are nothing else but the manifestations of the conflict that is going on within it on a level beyond the molecular.

"C. G. Jung noted that primitive people interpreted illness not as a weakness of the conscious mind but rather an inordinate strength of the unconscious mind in the process of transforming an individual from one stage of life to another. Symptoms may be the indication of an individual's attempt to undergo a profound self-healing process which may be disrupted rather than enhanced by chemotherapy."[9]

"Dermatitis, inflammation of the nerve ends of the skin, is often found to have a regenerative effect and may very well have its origin in some reactions of the defense mechanisms of the organism. **A seeming mishap may have the function of averting a catastrophe.**

"... we may get a statistical answer indicating to what extent epileptic seizures may be a necessity for this or that degree of complexity of combination among the myriad million units of our Olympian nerve-net, considering that whenever two or three nerve cells are gathered together a seizure may occur."[10]

The pattern of signs and symptoms will indicate the line of **least resistance** with which the defence system has chosen to best defend the organism.

For example, if an organism is already under stress due to a sexually transmitted disease, e.g. syphilis or gonorrhea, in order to abolish its symptoms medical treatment would call for a powerful drug to be prescribed and inserted into the chemistry of an already-stressed system. The organism's defenses, especially the immune system, will suffer a tremendous blow and a confused state will ensue. Under such stress its line of defense may start breaking down and a new "health condition" much worse than the previous one will be established.

According to the *Model* advanced here, AIDS is nothing but the result of constant and haphazard use of antibiotics, especially penicillin, on organisms already under extreme stress from previous exposures to infections (usually sexually transmitted diseases). At a certain point, the immune system is unable to counteract the constant inflow of chemicals and allows the disorder to manifest on a deeper level.

Using strong chemical agents (drugs) to counteract disease processes in human organisms already under stress, and not allowing enough time for recuperation from the previous use of chemicals, is analogous to breaking down the natural barriers of the system and promoting the degeneration of the human organism by producing **new** situations that will breed new "diseases."

"A modest course of antibiotics can disrupt surface body flora sufficiently to change body odors, vaginal secretions, and the ecology of skin. Diarrhea occurs in as many as one in every 8-10 patients after some antibiotics, a reflection of the damage done internally to the normal intestinal bacteria."[4]

"Extended broad-spectrum therapy is likely to induce candidiasis due to disruption of the normal ecologic balance of the intestinal flora."[11]

Today we in the West have arrived at an impossible situation where large numbers of people can face life only with a handful of medicine, taken every morning and night. Every day there is an obligatory intake of some kind of medicine to continue the process of living. We had better take the time now to consider just what it is that we have brought about, what it is that we have done to ourselves and, if we intend to continue as a human race, what it is that we have to do in the future. All those in positions of responsibility should pause to consider just what is happening. One would have hoped the AIDS situation would have given some food for thought to those in authority and thus provided the impetus for some long-awaited action on their part.

According to the *Model* presented here, the allopathic method of treatment does not usually promote health but rather, in many cases, promotes the rapid and aggressive deterioration of the organism. If we continue as we have been, we are going to bring about even worse conditions than AIDS and cancer.

It may appear that nothing could be worse than the pandemic of AIDS, but in truth the potential remains for serious affection to arise on even more profound levels of the human organism; I refer to the spiritual being, intellect and emotions. We have to be aware of such negative potentials, especially when it will soon be affecting very large percentage of the population; according to data published in 1986 "it is believed that there are 1.5 to 2 million AIDS carriers in the United States, while in Europe the numbers range from 250,000 to 500,000." But it can become much worse: "It is calculated that in every 8.8 months we will have a doubling of the population of AIDS carriers."[12]

At this point established medicine could ask, "What is the alternative treatment for venereal diseases, if not penicillin?" The answer is quite complex and the issue sufficiently broad in scope as to justify more than an offhand answer. But one's immediate reaction could be:

1. The public should be informed through the various means of mass communication that being infected with syphilis or gonorrhea is not the same as coming down with a common cold, and that simply taking penicillin does not eliminate the problem.

2. Even though the public is informed, there are still people who will contract syphilis or gonorrhea. These people's infections should be treated as something very serious, and if penicillin is prescribed, special care, attention and support should be given to the immune system with alternative methods of treatment, especially Homeopathy, until the patient has completely recovered.

3. The patient should be informed that in order to give his immune system enough time to completely recover from the shock of the disease and treatment, under no circumstances should he be reinfected within the next three years.

4. Research should be undertaken to establish precisely the different uses and possibilities of Homeopathy, Acupuncture and other alternative venues in treating such diseases. If the claims of the early homeopaths who treated syphilis hold true, then this form of treatment should be the first tried, and only if it fails should the physician resort to penicillin. In this way many people may be spared the destructive side effects of this powerful drug.

It is not the purpose of this treatise to discuss different alternative options or possibilities as solutions to the health problem. The issue is too broad and complicated to be discussed here. But what I would like to point out now is that what is needed in order to find a solution to the health problem is the adoption of a "correct attitude" on the part of the medical establishment. What is required as a first step is a change in attitude; the next step can then follow naturally.

REFERENCES:

1. Refer to references for Chapter 12 of this book.
2. THORNTON RC: *New Conceptions in Nuclear Physics.* GALLIMORE JG, *The Handbook of Unusual Energies.* California: Health Research, 1976
3. BLUMBERG BS: Australia antigen and the biology of hepatitis B. *Science 1977; 197: 17-25*
4. LAPPÉ M: *When Antibiotics Fail.* Berkeley, California: North Atlantic Books, 1986
5. EINSTEIN A: *The Principle of Relativity.* New York: Dover, 1923
6. SILVERMAN M, LEE PR: *Pills, Profits & Politics.* Berkeley: University of California Press, 1974
7. BRAITHWAITE J: *Corporate Crime in the Pharmaceutical Industry.* London: Routledge & Kegan Paul, 1984
8. MENNINGER K: *The Vital Balance. The Life Process in Mental Health and Illness.* New York: Viking Press, 1975
9. PELLETIER KR: *Mind as Healer, Mind as Slayer.* New York: Delacorte Press/Seymour Lawrence, 1977
10. WALTER WG: *The Living Brain.* WW Norton & Company, 1963
11. MARTIN EW: *Hazards of Medication.* Philadelphia, Toronto: JB Lippincott Company, 1971
12. PAPAEVANGELOU G: *AIDS* (Translation). Litsas, Athens: Medical Publications, 1986

Chapter 16

THE CONCEPT OF REGENERATION-DEGENERATION

35. Universal energy is "qualified" or modified by its passage through the mental, emotional and physical planes and is affected by the "data" (inherent predispositions) of each plane.

In a way, we have to imagine that the energy which animates the "triplex" (the mental, emotional and physical planes) of our being passes through the different planes of existence and is "colored" by the qualities of each level, which are unique for every individual. In the healthy state there is a harmonious flow of this energy passing through the levels, undispersed and undisturbed.

Thus we see that disease can be defined as **areas of restriction or knots of energy** that do not permit a harmonious flow of this force. Acupuncture therapy is actually based on this idea; through manipulation of the energy junctions (where energy bundles are supposedly located), it reestablishes the harmonious flow.

The three planes may generate and degenerate independently from each other. The decisive factor is where most of the knots are found. If they are on the physical level they will degenerate the physical part, if on the emotional level, the emotional part, and so forth.

The physician should keep in mind that two forces act upon the organism at all times. One tends to degeneration, dispersion and finally death. This is akin to the law of nature called entropy. The other is the force of life, that formative intelligence which promotes and gives form to all animate and inanimate manifestations on earth. These opposing forces are in constant motion keeping one another in check, balancing each other, as long as the individual remains alive. In the final outcome, for the physical body at least, entropy will prevail, and the physical body will disintegrate to its elemental constituents.

If the above holds true, we can logically deduce that the life principle should also prevail in some aspect since there has to be a balance between the two opposing forces. If indeed this is the case, the life principle will give the spiritual-psychic entity of the human being the possibility to survive, perhaps in another dimension.

If this is really a possibility, the only way that an individual may "survive" is to evolve spiritually and psychically by attaining a degree of perfection in those levels characterized by love and wisdom. In this way he will form an integrated and cohesive unit with very few separative-conflicting energies, and may thus remain a unified entity once out of the physical body. As we have mentioned before, the organization and perfection of these levels depend primarily on the conscious efforts of the individual.

If there remained a lot of negative energies (qualities) on the psychic, mental and spiritual planes at the time of death, our thought processes would be scattered and our emotional state confused at these final moments and therefore, we would be unable to realize the idea of a unified entity.

36. The more evolved a human being is, the more organized and coherent is the structure of his inner emotional and mental planes.

The evolution we are talking about here does not include or require sophisticated intellectual or scientific knowledge but rather real wisdom in understanding things in their essence, and thus the ability to work with nature rather than against it.

In order for the individual to evolve, he need not have a modern education. Having an education in modern societies can be an impediment rather than an asset. For example, an uneducated, simple or primitive person could give you a straightforward answer to a vital issue of pure ethics or conduct, whereas an educated person might give you an elaborate or confusing reply that he himself cannot comprehend.

37. Real changes in consciousness mark the evolutionary process of a human being. These changes do not

evolve as a smooth progressive process, but rather as jumps and leaps, reminding one of a quantum jump.

After a long period of conscious effort, one suddenly feels that he has attained better organization of his mental and emotional planes.

During certain times and under certain circumstances, the organism reaches "maximum organizational coherence." This may involve a conscious or unconscious effort on the part of the individual. At this given moment we have a sudden transition from a state of lower consciousness to a higher one. This also includes a new, higher, more sensitive state of emotions. What this means is that the organism has gathered more energy, more wisdom, to enter a higher state of consciousness—a higher energy level. In order to do this the organism is like an electron which needs a certain amount of "quanta" to go to an orbit of higher energy. The transition therefore is not a progressive one but a sudden one, akin to the nature of a **quantum jump**.

This idea is exemplified in the movement for "spiritual awareness" prevailing in our times. According to popular thought, people, given proper and thorough preparation, can quite "suddenly" enter a "new state of consciousness."

The fact that a human being uses only a very small portion of his brain in everyday life shows the almost infinite possibilities that exist in quantum jumps in consciousness and informational coherence or **Teleosis***. These jumps should not be viewed as physical achievements of the brain but rather as conscious and subconscious milestones of a self-directed evolutional process of the whole person.

38. **There are inherent tendencies within every human being to either attain a state of "Teleosis" ("synthesis," "maturity") or succumb to the law of entropy and "aposynthesis."**

Teleosis is not only a spiritual need but a universal urge that all human beings share and exhibit in whatever endeavor they attempt. Nobody who is healthy wants to be the worst in any particular activity he undertakes; on the contrary, he wants to be the best, the most perfect. This urge is very deeply entrenched in us. The area in which every individual wants to excel is not necessarily his profession; it can be the raising of his children or his hobby, etc. The fact remains that an individual who is healthy enough in the deeper levels needs to feel good about at least some of his activities; such aspirations for near-perfection include activities that range from the most basic to the most sublime and spiritual. This inner urge for perfection and attainment in every human being is what we call the "**law of Teleosis.**"

The reason that we have this urge is to overcome death or entropy. In different ways we try to make a "mark" in life so that our presence can remain forever in the memory of the living. This, in short, is the objective of Teleosis.

The more evolved an individual becomes, the more he aspires to do his best and be as "perfect" as possible in matters of a spiritual nature, and the less his interest is focused on "material" gain. Therefore we see that what is important for human beings is a state of Teleosis, where a sense of completeness, wholeness, maturity and happiness are the principal attainments. Nobody actually aspires to unhappiness, imperfection, destruction and entropy. Yet we should not forget that both these forces, entropy and Teleosis, are operating within us. This whole process of Teleosis is therefore closely connected with one's state of health.

Teleosis is promoted through:

A. **Conscious efforts** on the part of the individual to overcome weaknesses, negative thoughts and feelings, imperfections, barriers and obstructions.

B. **Efforts of a non-perceptible nature** of the organism to counteract minor stresses and stimulations that tend to disorganize it. (The organism is constantly busy bringing about the necessary subliminal changes to counteract minor stresses.)

C. **Efforts of the defense mechanism** that are mobilized under excessive stress to abort disaster (in which case we witness the development of signs and symptoms of disease).

The issues each individual organism will have to deal with concerning its health status are unique in their entirety and complexity.

In the physical body, the specific type of bacteria, virus, microbe, fungus, etc., that the organism attracts corresponds to the areas of weakness inherent in that particular physical organism and indicates the type of defense it will have to mobilize.

Conscious efforts to mobilize a defense against "aposynthesis" must be directed to correcting weaknesses of character, choosing paths that generate emotional well-being rather than upheaval, and cultivating mental-spiritual pursuits that improve the mind in all of its dimensions: subconscious, conscious and superconscious.

---

* **Teleosis** is a process by which a human being becomes more and more organized in his spiritual and psychic levels. He does this through a conscious effort that generates a series of changes bringing the individual closer and closer to a "perfect" state.

Chapter 17

DIRECTION OF DISORDER

39. The defense mechanism always has a built-in centrifugal tendency to keep disorder on the periphery (mucous membranes, skin), while a negative stressor has the opposite—a centripetal tendency—and thus pushes the disturbance to the center of the organism *(Figures 24 and 25).*

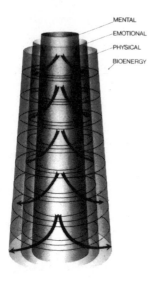

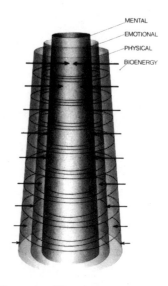

Figure 24: The organism will always tend to push the disorder to the periphery.

Figure 25: Negative stimulus tends to push the disorder towards more central or deeper organs or levels.

This mechanism is very important for the organism because it automatically evaluates the levels, systems and organs, and always tries to keep the disturbance in systems and organs that are more peripheral and therefore less important for the survival of the organism.

Evaluation of the human structure by the defense mechanism is amazing in complexity; even the most brilliant scientific mind cannot conceive its true dimension and meaning. In its evaluation the organism gives primary importance to the mental-spiritual plane and next to the emotional-psychic levels; consequently, the tendency of the defense mechanism is to protect these levels first from any possible disturbance. The organism will not allow a disturbance to easily manifest on these levels.

In spite of this logical evaluation by nature itself, these components of human existence have been the least understood by the logical, scientific, medical mind. They have been either unappreciated or appreciated for the wrong reasons and on the whole, they have largely been ignored. It is only when pain and suffering are present on these levels that we become aware of their existence and understand that they are actually very important components of our being. It is a well-known fact, attested to by many, that emotional suffering is unbearable and much worse than physical pain. Actually very few suicides have been committed because of physical pain. Most of these desperate, final acts have been undertaken because of emotional or mental suffering.

40. If stimulated properly (curatively), the organism will always tend to reorganize itself on all its planes and levels. If it cannot attain a "total cure," then it will tend to first heal its deeper and more essential parts and then proceed to the less essential and peripheral parts of its structure.

According to cybernetic laws, the organism will never heal an inflamed joint (peripheral part) if this leads to the detriment of more central parts or functions. Thus when strong anti-inflammatory drugs such as corticosteroids are used on an inflamed joint, much more serious symptoms appear in deeper, more important areas of the organism. In a really curative procedure, where the right kind of stimulation (therapy) has been applied, the organism will try to push the disorder into more peripheral areas, while at the same time relieving the central parts. It will do the opposite if the stimulation is wrong or suppressive, e.g. chemotherapy, corticosteroids, etc. This is another important fact relating directly to our health that has been totally ignored by established medicine.

Thus when a disease on the periphery like a skin eruption, colitis or an arthritic condition is given the wrong treatment, it retreats to the more essential organs or the deeper emotional and mental planes. In such circumstances the explanation given by the attending physician to the patient is usually, "Your suffering is psychological and has nothing to do with the treatment you received for your arthritis or skin eruption, etc. I can do nothing more for you. If you'd like I'll recommend a good psychiatrist." Eventually everybody has to see a psychiatrist!

Such a state of affairs is attributed, to a great extent, to our way of living rather than to the inner ecological imbalance resulting from the massive use of powerful allopathic drugs.

In reality the "new disturbance" (e.g. depression) on the mental or emotional plane is nothing other than the same arthritis or skin eruption pushed into the deeper levels of the organism, and which, at this point, has simply changed its form of expression.

If the organism receives the correct treatment later, the "depression" will disappear and the skin eruption or arthritis will reappear. This simple knowledge could save humanity a lot of suffering, yet the concept has never been mentioned or taught in medical schools.

41. Various levels of health exist between the ideal state of perfect health and the state of total deterioration. At this moment we are not certain about the number of levels existing between these two extremes, but for argument's sake we will list twelve of them.

The organism is at all times in a state of vibrating fluctuation but nevertheless remains within the limits of one of these levels. This state of vibrant fluctuation can be called a "hesitant state" because within it are contained many different probabilities. These probabilities give the organism the ability to remain in the lower or higher regions of the levels or to jump to a different level depending on the information or misinformation it receives.

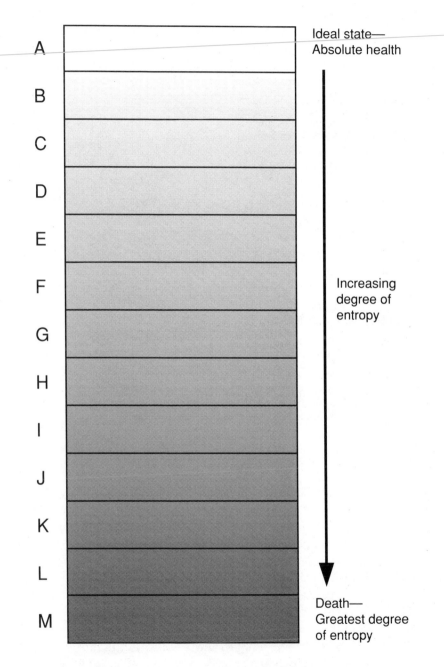

Figure 26: Differential health states of the organism.

The natural, healthy tendency of the organism is to stay in the higher regions of its level unless it is stressed. If it is stressed with a transient stressor it may drop to the lower or lowest regions of its present level.

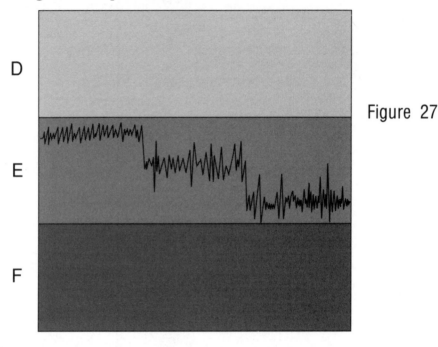

Figure 27

Figure 27: An organism which is at level "E" will tend to move up and down within its own level if the stressor is only mild.

But if it is stressed further by a stronger stressor, it may drop to another level altogether, which is lower in hierarchy.

This chronic disease state has always been marked by a quantum jump or essential change in energy patterns within the organism.

An example of this is an individual suffering from a common cold or influenza; as long as the cold lasts he feels pretty bad and his general state of health seems to drop, but his general chronic condition will not change and he will be back to his "pre-cold" state after the cold ends. If the acute condition is more serious, he will reach the lowest regions of his level and then subsequently return to the upper regions, once his recovery is complete. The same process may take place to a greater or lesser degree if one experiences a transient stress on the emotional and mental levels.

If, however, a person is already in a very sensitive condition because of an acute disease (transient stress) and receives

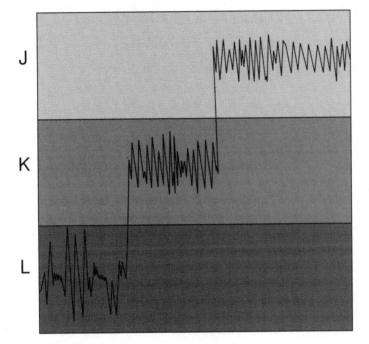

Figure 28

Figure 28: If the stressor is strong, the organism will jump to a lower level "L"; if proper treatment is given, it can jump to a higher level "J".

strong stress such as allopathic treatment, this will further stress his organism and possibly result in dropping him to a lower level altogether. To make this clearer, let us say someone was suffering from acute bronchitis and after the treatment a permanent asthmatic condition developed. Then the health of the whole organism would have been degraded one level. In this case the individual would remain permanently at this new level unless he received proper treatment. In a less fortunate situation he may be stressed even further, and even though his asthma disappears, he may descend to an even lower level where he develops a more serious condition like epilepsy, a severe heart condition or a mental problem.

Established medicine has never realized the continuity or connection between the different states of health in the individual because its theoretical perception deals only with diseases and their restricted connotation, rather than with diseased individuals.

42. The permanence of a negative (entropic) change (manifestation of a chronic disease) will depend on the intensity of the predisposition and that of the stressor, plus their corresponding mutual attraction.

In order for the organism to develop a chronic state, it needs to be deeply disturbed by a particular stress that bears a strong relation to the organism. In this case the whole organism drops to a lower level from which it cannot return through its own efforts. The organism now permanently resides on this level, and a chronic disease condition is established. This new chronic disease state has always been marked initially by a **quantum jump** or essential change in energy patterns within the organism.

In case the change is not permanent, the organism returns to its normal state within a few days or weeks; otherwise, the organism remains in its new chronic state without the possibility of self-recovery.

In other words, we can say that the organism will not fall permanently into a lower level unless it is stimulated by information or misinformation for which it has an extreme need or attraction.

A classical example of what has been stated is the immune reaction phenomenon following the use of a great variety of drugs such as aminopyrine, p-aminosalicylic acid, chlorpromazine, dipyrone, penicillin, chloramphenicol, a-methyldopa, some antineoplastics, etc.[1-4]

What clearly shows the importance of the intensity of the stressor is the fact that the repetitive use of these drugs results in an extreme immune response. An antigenic complex is formed which can induce the formation of specific antibodies against the drug. This demonstrates that the body's defense mechanism produces a reaction in order to allay the effects of these incoming drugs and to maintain its ecological balance.

43. As the organism changes levels of health, its predisposition to pathological agents changes accordingly.

Once an organism has dropped to another level of lower order there is a substantial change in its chemistry and whole energy structure. Different viruses or bacteria that previously thrived in an organism and affected it easily now do not affect it or affect it only with great difficulty. At the same time, the organism is now ready to be affected by new species of viruses, bacteria or fungi which this new physicochemical level attracts more easily. The new species that will now affect the organism are going to be of a more virulent nature and thus affect it more deeply and seriously. Because of the decrease in the resistance of the organism, even infecting agents that appear relatively harmless will for this organism be very virulent.

Finally, as the chronic disease processes progress deeper and become more centrally located in the organism, the emotional and mental planes are severely disturbed and the possibility of contracting an acute disease from a virus or bacteria is minimized. Thus the possibility of contracting an acute disease becomes inversely proportional to the severity of the mental or emotional disturbance. (The more severe the mental or emotional disturbance, the less chance of contracting an acute disease and vice versa.)

It is a well-known fact that in psychiatric wards severely disturbed mental patients seldom develop acute diseases. Autistic children or severely psychotic patients rarely if ever get infectious diseases. It is a common thing to hear an autistic child's mother say that the child never gets sick; that "he is so strong *otherwise.*" I never liked hearing this comment from mothers who brought in their children for treatment of mental disorders because it indicated the depth of their illness. Some observers believe that schizophrenics are oddly resistant to virus infections. A monumental study of mortality statistics in Russia, Greece, Scotland and Wales has disclosed that psychiatric patients are afflicted by cancer at less than one-third the rate of the general population. Schizophrenics are especially resistant to cancer.

The explanation for this phenomenon is probably that the blood chemistry of a mentally ill person becomes a very hostile environment for the recognized virus, bacteria or fungus.

According to this *Model*, the decrease in the number of people affected by infectious diseases and epidemics in the western world today is not only due to hygienic and sanitary measures but also to the fact that they **cannot** be infected due to the **decline of the general level of health.** The pathology of the population in general is so deep that it prevents the infectious diseases from taking hold and showing an increase in frequency. For instance, according to this *Model,* it will be almost impossible to infect a schizophrenic patient with AIDS no matter what quantity of the virus you inject into him. Furthermore, this *Model* suggests that if a severely disturbed mental patient were injected with the AIDS virus and then came down with the AIDS disease, the physical condition would automatically relieve his mental symptomatology.

44. It is quite difficult to discern whether bacteria, viruses or fungi have come from the outside environment or have developed endogenously due to certain specific internal conditions.

The question is whether microorganisms start multiplying at great speed once they have infected an organism with an environment conducive to their development, or whether the internal conditions of the organism have deteriorated to such a degree that these microorganisms are automatically produced by an endogenous process of mutation into new kinds of pathological viruses, bacteria or fungi.

The most probable hypothesis is that **both processes** can take place, with the critical parameter being the inner conditions of the organism or the degree of degeneration.

The idea that a virus or bacterium may mutate into another species which can be harmful to the organism is neither new nor unacceptable.[5] Pasteur's idea was that if the microbes and bacteria were killed the organism would be free of disease. This sounded plausible at the time, but diseases have not been eliminated even though this dictum has been followed rigorously.

"The period once euphemistically called the Age of the Miracle Drugs is dead. Only the most optimistic observers can believe that we stand much of a chance of recapturing the spirit and hope of that age of some forty years ago. And only the most short-sighted could hope to see a reconstruction of that wonderful era when we believed we were on the verge of chemically conquering all infectious diseases. **We tried, and the evolutionary prowess of the microbial world won out.**"[6]

During Pasteur's time there was another French scientist called Bechamp who proposed a theory exactly opposite that of Pasteur. Bechamp maintained that it was mainly the "soil" or condition of the host organism at the moment that determined whether or not an individual would fall ill. The world followed Pasteur because his theories appeared more "logical," while Bechamp's were rather peculiar and difficult to prove.

At this time, allopathic medicine was starting to establish itself as the main therapeutic modality in the world. When pharmaceutical companies joined the battle and exerted their power to influence medical doctors to prescribe their products exclusively, the supremacy of allopathy was virtually ensured. As a consequence, the ambitions and narrow-minded rhetoric of its institutions came to dominate the entire western medical world.

It is my belief that in the future the dictums of disease that allopathy imposes will prove not only wrong but disastrous for humanity. History will show that Pasteur, and with him the rest of the world, misinterpreted the phenomena he observed. Today the theories of Bechamp are being re-examined by several scientists. Their research is lending increased plausibility to his ideas.

At the beginning of this century, a little before the time of the dispute between the two French scientists Pasteur and Bechamp, an American physician called J. T. Kent wrote in his book *Lectures on Homeopathic Philosophy,* "The bacteria are results of disease. In the course of time we will be able to show perfectly that the microscopial little fellows are not the disease cause but that they come after, that they are scavengers accompanying the disease...."[7]

45. In order to stimulate therapeutically an organism suffering from chronic or acute disease, we either have to introduce "batches" of subtle energy corre-

sponding to the ones generated by the organism under stress, or harmonize and release the obstructed flow of universal energy. In either case the therapeutic stimulation is not only on a physicochemical level but on an energy level as well.

In this *Model of Health and Disease*, we have been dealing with an energy system rather than simply a material system. It is natural that we should think that the appropriate therapeutic method should be concerned with an energetic stimulation rather than a chemical one. What we have tried to show so far is that the ideal way of treating the human organism is not by chemical drugs which affect certain local areas of the immune system, but by stimulating the whole defense system of the organism on an energy level. The important thing to remember is that we have to **stimulate the organism in the same direction that it itself would use in combatting the disease**. Therefore, an appropriate treatment or therapy should be on an energy level and in the same direction that the organism itself has chosen for its defense.

Therefore, if we could provide energy waves that imitated the energy generated by the defense system, we could avoid all side effects while at the same time giving the best possible help to the natural defenses of the body. Does such an ideal therapeutic system exist? The answer is yes.

Homeopathy, a holistic system of therapy and an alternative modality to established medicine, is based entirely on this idea.[9] So far, this therapeutic modality has been neglected, disregarded or completely ignored by "mainstream medicine" and its adherents. A short exposition of this system will be given in later chapters.

46. **A cure takes place as a quantum jump and is composed of newly forming patterns of energy with greater coherence. Under the right stimulation the organism reaches a state of "informational optima" in a split second. After this occurs, physiological processes will take place over time.**

In the same way that disease occurs as an instant energy change, the organism will return to a normal state under the right energy stimulation with a quantum jump.

Even though the local suffering has changed very little or not at all, this quantum jump is experienced by the patient as a feeling of greater vitality, freedom and well-being.

If such a feeling emerges immediately after treatment, it is a sign that the cure for the local condition will soon come as well.

It is very important that this point is understood by all, since it is in this way that anyone under treatment is going to perceive whether the medicine is bringing about the desired effect. If, on the contrary, a treatment brings about a sense of discomfort, confusion, dissatisfaction and a general energy drop, it will mean that it is acting in a suppressive rather than in a curative manner.

47. Chronic disturbance or chronic disease has an underlying continuity which can be manifested at different levels, its symptomatology changing dramatically as the disturbance changes from one level to another. As the disturbance becomes more intense and locates more centrally in the organism, the level of health drops.

As an example, we have the case of a patient suffering from condylomata of the genitalia (a skin manifestation). The allopathic treatment relieves the patient of the condylomata but in a suppressive manner because the whole disturbance may now change into a chronic cystitis pattern (another level) which, in turn, if suppressed further, may develop into chronic ulcerative colitis. If the disturbance is pushed further into deeper regions, the colitis may eventually change into a severe anxiety state.

In such a case, the suffering will be greatest when the disease has been pushed to the mental and emotional planes and the patient develops anxiety. The least suffering will be felt when the patient is back to his original "condylomata" state.

When a real cure of the condylomata (after the initial disappearance) is achieved, there is no further chronic disease development in this organism, but rather a return to health.

It appears that almost no one within established medicine or society recognizes the fact that the development of chronic disease is neither accidental nor incidental, but is a strict, almost mathematical, sequence of events which many times originates from wrong treatment and the use of crude chemical drugs.

48. Just as the health of individuals displays continuity (e.g. in the manifest consequences of suppressive treatment), so does the course of human disease on the planet vary according to external circumstances. For instance, the appearance and predominance of certain diseases vary in relation to the degree of exposure of the human species to pollution, radiation, massive allopathic drugging, etc.

So, for instance, while we observe that during a specific period of time certain diseases decline and others increase, the overall result is that the intensity of disease in general remains on the ascendancy. While acute rheumatic fever and tuberculosis have declined, salmonellosis, chlamydia, non-specific urethritis, herpes, AIDS and a host of other new diseases have increased tremendously.

In earlier times, diseases that ravaged society were generally concerned with the lower levels of the physical-emotional-mental planes, on the periphery of such systems as the cardiovascular, genitourinary, nervous, etc. But as societies have developed, new diseases emerged that penetrate more deeply the levels of the different planes; and thus these diseases are far more devastating. Just as diseases evolve in an individual, so they obviously evolve on a global scale. Simple diseases have evolved into more complex and difficult ones. We have gone from dysentery, typhus and malaria to pneumonia and tuberculosis, and then to cardiovascular diseases, nervous disorders, cancer, schizophrenia and finally AIDS.

It is also interesting to note that diseases which have been prominent for several decades now display a resistance to treatment, making them much more difficult to manage (salmonellosis, gonorrhea, malaria, etc.).

In short, one can say that whenever we have tried interfering in an unwise manner with the organism's inner ecology by attacking its microorganisms, we have invariably won the battle and lost the war. Where we expected to eliminate disease, we have created new ones even more resistant, vicious and lethal.

For example, in developed countries (using the Federal Republic of Germany as an example), premature mortality rate due to malignant neoplasms (cancer) is much higher than in developing countries (using Mexico as an example). Ischaemic heart disease is quite prevalent in developed countries, while absent in developing countries. The same pattern holds for suicide rates, which appear significant only in developed countries. At the same time, premature mortality rate in developing countries from infectious disease is quite significant, while in developed countries it is insignificant.

REFERENCES:

1. THEIRFELDER von S, MAGIS C, SAINT-PAUL M, et al: "Die Puramidon-Agranulocytoze." *Dtsch Med Wschr 1964; 89: 506*
2. PARKER CW: *Drug Reaction in Immunological Diseases.* Boston: Little Brown and Co., 1965
3. McGIBBON BH, LONGBRIDGE LW, HOWIHANE DO, et al. Autoimmune Hemolytic Anemia with Acute Renal Failure due to Phenacetin and p-Aminosalicylic Acid. *Lancet, 1970; 1: 7-10*
4. MARTIN EW: *Hazards of Medication.* Philadelphia, Toronto: JB Lippincott Co., 1970
5. Reference in the introduction
6. LAPPÉ M: *When Antibiotics Fail.* Berkeley, California: North Atlantic Books, 1986
7. HUME ED: *Bechamp or Pasteur?* London: The CW Daniel Company, 1932
8. KENT JT: *Lectures on Homoeopathic Philosophy.* Berkeley: North Atlantic Books, 1980
9. VITHOULKAS G: *The Science of Homeopathy.* New York: Grove Press, Inc., 1980

Chapter 18

THE HYPOTHESIS ABOUT AIDS

As a logical conclusion to the preceding chapters, one can say that the state of AIDS has come about primarily because of the very treatment these individuals received for their frequent venereal infections.

Jaffe and colleagues reported that in case studies of homosexuals with AIDS, eighty-six percent had a history of gonorrhea and sixty-eight percent a history of syphilis.[1]

Yet these figures do not tell the whole story, since those suffering from asymptomatic gonococcal infections as well as pharyngeal gonococcal infections were not accounted for in the statistics. Since these cases comprise a large percentage of the total number of those infected with venereal diseases, the numbers given above would be much higher if they included these infections as well.

This point is exemplified in a study of homosexuals done in Los Angeles by Merino and Richards, where it was found that up to 70% of patients with anal gonococcal infections and 90% of patients with pharyngeal gonococcal infections were asymptomatic.[2]

A likely explanation is that after having a casual sexual contact, many homosexuals through their own initiative took antibiotics as a prophylactic measure in case they had contracted a venereal disease. If they had indeed contracted any venereal disease, what they were in effect doing was masking the symptoms by taking the antibiotics, and not really eliminating the pathogenic microorganism. (It is very unlikely that these individuals would have reported such incidents since it was probably too frequent an occurrence with them because of their lifestyle.) S. Landis, in a paper summarizing the occurrence of sexually transmitted diseases in Canada and the frequency of gonococcal infections within the homosexual population, suggests that this knowledge should have been enough of a reason for changing their sexual behavior.[3]

These facts have been confirmed by homosexual AIDS patients whom I have personally supervised and who have given me the history of their sexual practices. The figures sometimes ran to extremes, and some claimed to have had as many as one thousand sexual partners in one year. From such numerous encounters one can easily imagine the number of venereal infections which could occur.

So, when my students and I looked at the medical histories of these patients, we ascertained repeated incidences of venereal infection and, as a consequence, frequent and protracted courses of antibiotics. According to our estimation, the percentage of AIDS cases with several incidences of sexually transmitted diseases in their medical histories was greater than 90%.

Actually several researchers had already noted this fact but paid little attention to it or did not relate it in any particular way to the AIDS issue. The incidence of venereal infections in AIDS patients was so common that early researchers noticed it right away, as indicated in references 1 and 4 to 7.

It is of great importance to note that female homosexuals, although they might have been very active sexually, are not in the high-risk groups. The reason, according to this hypothesis, is that this group's type of sexual practice does not include "penetration" (actual coition). Thus, these women infrequently contracted sexually transmitted diseases and did not need frequent treatment with antibiotics.

If this hypothesis is right, several critical questions remain:

1. **If it were venereal disease coupled with antibiotic treatment that brought about the state of AIDS, why did we not witness this kind of epidemic earlier, since penicillin and other antibiotics have been the preferred prescription drugs for venereal disease for more than thirty years.**

The answer to this question is that repeated assaults with venereal diseases and repeated courses of antibiotics were probably needed before there was sufficient degradation of the organism's immune system to allow this opportunistic virus to emerge from within.

In addition, society's views on homosexuality fifteen to twenty years ago were much more conservative. Male homosexuals did not have the opportunity to freely indulge in sexual practices (communal baths, gay bars, etc.); therefore, the potential for frequent infections was much less.

It appears that most of the time the human organism has the ability to recuperate and regain its balance if it is not grossly damaged by repeated assaults with extreme drug doses. Some organisms will take longer to recuperate than others, and it is only a small percentage that will not recover from the assault if a drug-free period is allotted to re-establish balance. Due to repeated attacks of venereal infections, many homosexuals did not give their immune systems a chance to recuperate. An extensive explanation of this idea has already been given in the preceding chapters of this book.

2. How can we explain the fact that except for homosexuals and promiscuous heterosexuals, the next most highly involved AIDS group has been Haitians?

There has been some confusion concerning this issue because researchers tried to find a specific impediment in the Haitians' immune system that would account for the "high-risk" position of this group. The answer to this quandary according to my hypothesis seems to be much simpler than originally thought.

The largest male homosexual populations are located in San Francisco, Los Angeles and New York. As with all social groups with a religious, ethnic, or in this case, sexual preference, places arise that become the "in spots" for vacations. Haiti was the "in place" to go for many homosexuals. It was close to the U.S., relatively safe, cheap, provided sexual partners, had easy political access and was the ideal place for a casual sexual encounter.

As a result, these visitors infected a great number of the indigenous population with their venereal diseases and eventually with AIDS as well. In turn, the local population, including bisexuals, infected the prostitutes who in turn infected other men. All these people consequently had to take enormous amounts of antibiotics, and thereby a situation conducive for the development of the AIDS disease was created. It is at this point that we actually witness the proof of this theory.

In support of these ideas we cite the following excerpt from the research paper titled "The Acquired Immunodeficiency Syndrome in Haiti":

"The recognition of Kaposi's sarcoma and opportunistic infections in Haiti was temporally related to the appearance of AIDS in the United States. The earliest possible case of opportunistic infection in Haiti that is known to our group occurred in July 1978, and the first case of fulminant Kaposi's sarcoma was diagnosed in June 1979. The first cases of Kaposi's sarcoma and opportunistic infections in homosexual men in the United States were documented in early 1978 . We do not believe that AIDS was present in Haiti before 1978. This contention is supported by the clinical experience of the practicing pathologists and dermatologists in Haiti and by our inability to identify earlier cases through examination of autopsy and biopsy records."[8]

3. Why are prostitutes and promiscuous men the next high-risk group?

It is because they are exposed to frequent venereal infections and therefore prone to frequent courses of antibiotics.

4. Why is there an explosion of AIDS in Africa?

For the last ten to fifteen years, epidemics of syphilis and gonorrhea have affected unprecedented numbers of people in Africa. In the African countries it is often difficult to collect accurate data because many of these cases are either not reported or are "self-treated" with over-the-counter antibiotics. Despite this under-reporting, there are several countries in Africa where syphilis and gonococcal infections rank first or second in incidence among all infectious diseases. Furthermore, the number of people with sexually transmitted diseases is greater than all other infectious disease cases put together. This is startling information considering these countries have a great number of infectious diseases such as malaria, measles, parasitic infections, etc. The statistics of the World Health Organization (WHO) show that this is, in fact, the case in such countries as Botswana, French Territory of the Affars and Issas, Guinea-Bissau, Reunion, Senegal, Uganda, Gambia, Guinea, Lesotho, Mali, Mauritius, Morocco and the Seychelles.[9,10]

That congenital syphilis is so prevalent in these countries is also suggestive of the enormous venereal disease epidemic prevalent in Africa at the moment. The treatment of such diseases in Africa is far from standardized. Many of the local population who are infected take antibiotics over-the-counter for lack of availability of physicians, and probably overdose themselves to ward off infection.

One can now see the whole picture of repeated venereal infection in all these high-risk groups. The sexual liberation in Africa and the homosexual "revolution" in the West have brought about the same result—namely, frequent venereal infections and, consequently, repeated courses of antibiotics.

In Botswana in 1973, out of 608,654 inhabitants 28,204 had gonorrheal infections and 9,750 had syphilis.

In Chad, in a population of 3,254,000 in 1974, there were 5,035 cases of congenital syphilis, 9,222 cases of early syphilis, and 20,636 cases of gonococcal infections.

In Gabon, in a population of 448,564, there were 13,793 cases of gonococcal infections in 1973.

In Gambia, in a population of 487,448, the number of gonococcal infections was 6,391 in 1980.

In Guinea-Bissau, in a population of 487,448 in 1981, there were 5,829 cases of gonococcal infections.

In Mali, in a population of 6,035,272 in 1973, there were 32,993 cases of syphilis and 21,235 cases of gonococcal infections.

In Niger, in a population of 2,501,800 in 1981, there were 14,230 cases of congenital syphilis, 9,171 of syphilis, 30,255 of gonococcal infections, and 4,809 cases of other venereal diseases.

In Senegal, in a population of 5,085,388 in 1974, there were 1,063 cases of congenital syphilis, 6,680 cases of early syphilis, 58,144 cases of syphilis, and 18,678 cases of gonococcal infections.

In Sudan, in a population of 14,113,590 in 1979, there were 48,826 cases of early syphilis and 56,202 cases of gonococcal infections.

In Uganda, in a population of 9,548,847 in 1974, there were 9,660 cases of syphilis and 331,992 cases of gonococcal infections.

In Zaire in 1973, 1,407 cases of congenital syphilis, 5,234 cases of early syphilis, 9,829 cases of syphilis, and 126,224 cases of gonococcal infections were reported. [9,10]

According to this *Model,* countries where religious, social and ethical morals are still strong will be less affected by this epidemic.

The question remains, is it axiomatic that a person who has undergone treatment for syphilis or gonorrhea and has taken a lot of antibiotics in his past will contract AIDS or become an

AIDS carrier once exposed? The answer is NO. What I suggest is that **a compromised immune system of a particular order** will lead to AIDS, and the easiest way to bring about such a state is by having frequent venereal infections followed by repeated antibiotic treatment.

5. Why are drug users a high-risk group?

First of all, one has to take into consideration that many drug users also belong to the high-risk group of homosexuals, and this causes some confusion. On the other hand, daily drug use weakens the organism's immune system and prepares it to accept the virus more readily, once introduced through use of an infected needle.

Drug users were actually the "secondary" victims of the epidemic. The previous groups could develop the virus through an endogenous process, while this group "prepared" its members to become prospective victims of the disease through the exogenous route.

Factors that promote degeneration by compromising the immune system

According to my hypothesis, an organism is ready to admit the virus and provide a conducive environment once it has reached a "critical point" in its inner balance, or in this case "imbalance." This imbalance can result from the assault of the organism by different agents, such as the following:

A. All strong allopathic drugs, especially those which have a direct impact on the immune system like antibiotics, antihistamines, antifungal agents, corticosteroids, chemotherapeutic drugs, etc., given repeatedly and in high dosages, can bring the organism to an AIDS-developing state. The human organism can usually tolerate small amounts of such drugs and will reestablish its balance automatically by its natural adaptability; but very few constitutions exist today which can tolerate long and repeated courses of such strong drugs without dire consequences.

Another problem is the passing of a predisposition from parents to children. Once the parents' immune systems are compromised, a child born to these parents will have the weakness-predisposition passed on to them. They will be at high risk for developing the virus. Because they already have a predisposition, such children do not have to receive immunosuppressive treatments during their lifetime in order to develop the disease. This is the reason why we are going to see more and more cases of children developing AIDS.

B. The next big factor which appears to play an important role in compromising the immune system is illicit, non-prescription drug use—LSD, cocaine, morphine, heroin, etc. These drugs by their very nature create a physical or psychological dependence and therefore are used on an increasingly frequent basis. Again in this case, the organism is not given enough time to recuperate between assaults, and the additive effect of each new dose of the drug is magnified enormously, causing the immune system's final breakdown.

C. The organism is further stressed by environmental factors such as air pollution, industrial waste and automobile exhaust fumes, etc.

D. It is also stressed from food preservatives and other chemicals used today for the production of food, fertilizers, disinfectant spays, etc.

E. Radiation in the atmosphere from nuclear accidents and atomic weapons tests adds to the stress.

F. There is anxiety, grief and stress due to the competitive climate prevalent in our societies today.

G. Lack of proper nutrition also compromises immune competence.

High-risk individuals

In order for an individual to develop AIDS, he will need a certain degree of predisposition. Such a condition is either genetic or can be developed during his lifetime through specific stresses. It is the degree of susceptibility which will predispose some people to be carriers of the virus with little or no signs of the disease, others to be infected and develop AIDS symptoms in ten to fifteen years from the date of infection, and still others to develop severe AIDS symptoms soon after becoming exposed to the virus.

According to this *Model* the highest risk groups in order are:

A. Individuals who have had repeated exposures to venereal disease and frequent antibiotic treatments, and who also have a genetic predisposition towards this kind of infection. Even if there is no evidence at this time that such a predisposition exists, I believe that in the very near future it will be made evident by research.

These individuals have the greatest risk because their immune systems have suffered the greatest damage. While checking the past medical history of such individuals, we find that antibiotics were not only taken as treatment for confirmed infections, but also as precautionary measures after risky contacts.

B. People who have taken a lot of prescription and non-prescription drugs.
C. Those whose health has been degraded by frequent diseases, especially with hepatitis type-B virus and other acute diseases.

Low-risk individuals
A. Those who exhibit excellent health relatively untouched by drugs, pollution and food preservatives. Such individuals may be found in remote areas of the world, usually inaccessible high mountainous regions which do not have much contact with today's "high-tech civilization." For example, such people can be found in South America, the Caucasus, India, Pakistan and Africa, among other places.
B. The chronically ill who suffer from diseases our modern societies have produced such as Alzheimer's dementia and other serious mental disorders. These are chronic diseases which have to do with the central nervous system.

Also included are schizophrenics confined to mental institutions, severe cases of epilepsy, diabetics in advanced stages, those with systemic diseases like lupus erythematosus and cancer in its last stage, etc. This group of people is probably protected because of their chronic disease condition which taken as a whole is a greater hazard than AIDS.

Factors promoting the degeneration of the human body
It is a big mistake on our part to attribute the consequences of thirty to forty years of violations to the ecology of the human organism on AIDS. According to this *Model*, the modern-age explosion of severe, degenerative, chronic diseases like cancer, Alzheimer's disease, multiple sclerosis, neuromuscular disor-

ders and systemic diseases, results from a degeneration related to frequent and excessive use of allopathic drugs and vaccinations.

How else can one explain the tremendous increase in degenerative diseases in the West as compared to underdeveloped or developing countries that have not yet seen the menace of these diseases?

Cancer (neoplasms) account for roughly twice as many deaths in the developed countries as in developing countries and for about one-tenth of the total mortality rate; they account for 19% of the deaths in the developed countries and only 6% of deaths in the developing countries.

50% of the deaths in Europe are estimated to occur from diseases of the circulatory system and certain degenerative diseases, and a further 17% of deaths are due to neoplasms.

It is more than obvious from the statistics* compiled by the World Health Organization (WHO) that developed countries like the U.S., Canada, Belgium and England have a cancer mortality rate ranging from 13% to 16%, while the underdeveloped countries like El Salvador, Honduras, Peru, etc., have a rate ranging between 3% and 5%. As countries "develop" and make "better health coverage" accessible, the percentage of degeneration increases. One may tend to attribute such degenerative diseases to the anxiety and stress produced by modern technology in our lives. This is not true as seen from the mortality statistics of Western Communist countries where it is known that there is far less anxiety from competition since everyone's source of livelihood is virtually assured by the government.

*Statistics of death rates from cancer in percentages[11,12,13]

	1979	1980	1981	1982	1983	1984	1985
Developed countries:							
Scotland					16.08	16.09	16.08
Belgium	15.40			15.40		15.30	
England/ Wales				14.53		15.08	
Canada	13.20	13.20	13.09	13.60			
USA		13.10		13.10	13.22		
Austria				13.90	13.70		13.45
France			13.90	13.90		13.95	
FDR				13.92		13.60	
Italy	13.54	13.58	13.50				

	1981	1982	1983	1984	1985
Communist bloc countries:					
Hungary		16.59		16.75	16.65
Czechoslovakia	15.78		16.14	16.23	
Developing countries:					
Honduras	3.14				
El Salvador			3.39		
Dominican Republic		5.18			
Peru		5.84			
Mexico		7.18			
Mauritius	8.34				7.18
Panama			7.60	7.80	
Puerto Rico		7.87	9.39		

Actually, the populations of communist countries are known for their lack of anxiety and their sense of boredom, as well as for their low productive output. But it is also a fact that they do have extensive health coverage. I am positive that if an in-depth survey is done in these countries, it will be found that many people go to the medical doctors in order to get sick leave from work; consequently, the physicians are forced to prescribe drugs for them. Maybe this is the reason why these countries have the highest rates of degenerative diseases, even higher than their "free-world" counterparts.

Another disease that has appeared lately as a classic example of a degenerative disorder of the mental plane is **Alzheimer's disease.**

"It has been reported that about 4.4% of people over 65 display moderate to severe senile dementia, and that about 65% of these have Alzheimer's disease: a prevalence rate greater than three per 1,000 of the whole population. Since the life expectancy of these patients is much reduced, over 100,000 deaths per year may be related to Alzheimer's disease in the elderly." [14]

"Estimates of the incidence of Alzheimer's among patients over age 65 with organic dementia vary between 40% and 58%. Applying these figures to the United States, the prevalence of Alzheimer's disease in persons over 65 would be between 350,000 and 510,000 in 1970.

"The prevalence of severe dementia or organic psychosis, terms used to describe patients in whom, in addition to an intellectual deterioration, there was evidence of disorganization of the personality and inability to carry out the normal tasks of daily living, averaged 4.1%. Between 60,000 and 90,000 persons with senile dementia die each year, and these estimates do not take into account persons under age 65 or those within whom the moderate forms of dementia shorten the life expectancy. This estimate of the prevalence of Alzheimer's disease has been based on conservative assumptions." [15]

By far, the disease that appears to be almost exclusively a stigma of the "developed" countries is multiple sclerosis.

"No well-documented case of multiple sclerosis has ever been reported in African blacks." [16]

However, the prevalence of multiple sclerosis among immigrants to the Republic of South Africa from United Kingdom and other parts of northern and central Europe was approximately 49 per 100,000 population. In a study showing the local epidemiology of the disease, the areas in which it appears most prevalent (high-risk zones) include Northern Europe, North America and Southern Canada. What better example could we have than this? It actually shows us that well-developed countries, countries in which the human organism has been manipulated with myriad drugs and vaccinations, are now having serious health problems.

It is my suspicion that multiple sclerosis is the result of vaccination. Countries where vaccination was introduced long ago have a very high incidence of multiple sclerosis, whereas in Arab and African countries, which did not introduce vaccination as early, we find almost no incidence of multiple sclerosis.

Alter, studying the immigrants and native-born Jewish populations of Israel, noted that while the disease was rare among the native Israelis and immigrants from other Near East countries and North Africa, it is considerably more prevalent among immigrants from Central Europe, and was even more frequent among those from Northern Europe. Further study of immigration data revealed that age at immigration appeared to play an extremely important role. A person leaving his country of origin before the age of 15 years would have a risk of acquiring multiple sclerosis similar to that of the native-born Israeli or South African; an individual immigrating after that age would carry with him the risk factor of his country of origin. Another study demonstrated a major difference in the prevalence of multiple sclerosis among Afro-Asian immigrants and their Israeli-born offspring. In the latter group, there was a twofold increase in prevalence within just one generation. Thus native-born Israelis of either European or Afro-Asian origin now have prevalence rates of multiple sclerosis as high as the European immigrants. [16-22]

Here is some population data showing the extent of the problem:

Between 1957 and 1970 there were only two patients who may have been cases of multiple sclerosis in Nigeria.
In Ghana multiple sclerosis did not occur before 1970.
In Kenya only two patients with multiple sclerosis had been seen between 1952 and 1969.
Multiple sclerosis has not been diagnosed in any African in Bulawayo, although it has been seen in Rhodesian-born whites.[17]
In contradistinction, in Canada in 1973 there were 211 patients and 204 patients in1976.

Multiple sclerosis	1972	1973	1974	1977	1978
Developed countries:					
USA	1704			1372	
Austria		109	121		91
Denmark					1964
FDR					849
Netherlands					135
Norway					43
Sweden					92
Switzerland					110
Scotland					101
Communist bloc countries:					
Hungary					99
Poland				507	512
Developing countries:					
Egypt	0				
Mauritius		0	0		0
Barbados		0		0	
Costa Rica				0	
Surinam		1			
Trinidad		0			
Singapore		0			

9.23

Degenerative diseases of the circulatory system

Half of those who die in the European countries and 32% of deaths in the Western Pacific Region succumb to diseases of the circulatory system.

The chances of dying from cerebrovascular diseases and all other diseases of the circulatory system (at age 45) are respectively

	Death from cerebrovascular diseases	Death from other diseases of circulatory system	Year
Developed countries:			
Canada	7.82%	42.50%	1982
USA	7.00%	45.30%	1983
Austria	14.56%	38.35%	1985
France	10.27%	25.54%	1984
FDR	11.05%	39.36%	1985
Italy	13.01%	34.57%	1981
Sweden	8.80%	48.50%	1983
Communist bloc countries:			
Bulgaria	21.95%	39.35%	1984
Czechoslovakia	14.68%	39.54%	1984
Hungary	15.09%	38.37%	1985
Romania	14.91%	47.17%	1984
Developing countries:			
Sri Lanka	2.75%	18.18%	1980
Kuwait	3.37%	38.77%	1982
El Salvador	4.56%	12.74%	1983
Honduras	5.12%	13.97%	1981

Death rates due to diseases of the circulatory system:

Developed countries:		
Canada	33.96%	1984
USA	40.77%	1983
Austria	46.88%	1984
France	26.24%	1984
FDR	41.71%	1985
Sweden	39.40%	1984
Northern Ireland	50.00%	1985
Scotland	50.52%	1985
Communist bloc countries:		
Hungary	68.10%	1985
Bulgaria	66.54%	1984
Czechoslovakia	65.78%	1984
Romania	76.24%	1984
Developing countries:		
Costa Rica	15.23%	1983
Dominican Republic	16.00%	1982
El Salvador	10.63%	1983
Honduras	11.64%	1981
Mexico	17.25%	1982
Peru	12.00%	1982

11.12.13

WHO Region		Estimated population in 1980	Estimated no. of deaths (in thousands) from:						Estimated number of deaths (in 1,000's) at age:				Total (in 1,000's)
									0–14	15–44	45–64	65+	
AFR	Africa	380.895	3.566	206	836	613	270	1.675	4.409	1.150	734	873	7.166
AMR	America	608.717	1.057	729	1.908	288	373	876	1.366	608	971	2.286	5.231
DVG	Developing	251.758	981	282	773	263	198	653	1.294	440	511	905	3.150
DVD	Developed	356.959	76	447	1.135	25	175	223	72	168	461	1.380	2.081
SEA	S. E. Asia	1.050.726	6.777	672	2.407	1.282	660	3.634	8.062	1.998	2.552	2.820	15.432
EUR	Europe	813.573	971	1.444	4.297	207	487	1.105	860	565	1.471	5.615	8.511
DVG	Developing	64.518	310	47	149	70	38	185	406	81	110	202	799
DVD	Developed	749.055	661	1.397	4.148	137	449	920	454	484	1.361	5.413	7.712
EM	E. Medit.	267.412	1.762	165	559	386	163	927	2.387	420	459	686	3.962
WP	W. Pacific	1.308.017	2.691	1.026	3.315	473	712	2.265	1.871	1.524	2.797	4.290	10.482
DVG	Developing	1.173.428	2.623	829	2.890	466	649	2.167	1.846	1.463	2.620	3.695	9.624
DVD	Developed	134.589	68	197	425	7	63	98	26	61	176	595	858
TOT	World total	4.438.338	16.824	4.242	13.322	3.249	2.665	10.482	18.965	6.265	8.984	16.570	50.784

Infectious and parasitic diseases including certain respiratory diseases

Neoplasms

Diseases of circulatory system and certain degenerative diseses

Certain diseases originating in the perinatal period

Injury and poisoning

All other and unknown causes

Figure 29: Deaths by cause and age, WHO Regions, 1980.

While it is true that a genetic predisposition exists in everyone, that predisposition may never manifest itself unless there is a major assault to the immune system. What is really frightening is the possibility that these drugs and vaccinations may so undermine the immune system that they will cause genetic mutations to be transmitted from parents to the next generation.

I do not want to denigrate the importance of other factors in the degeneration of the human race, but experience has shown us that all other factors combined are nothing in comparison with the immediate and deep damage that allopathic drugs wreak upon the body's ecology. What Ivan Illich wrote 10 years ago in his book *Medical Nemesis* becomes almost prophetic today: **"the gravest health hazard we face today is our medical system."** Yet lay people and the medical establishment in general have virtually ignored his well-researched book.

Many other researchers and scientists such as Dubos, Mendelsohn, Gardner, Weitz, Silverman, Lee, Menninger, Ferguson, Lappé, McKeown, Klass and Pelletier joined their voices to warn the public that the storm was approaching with great speed, but no one with authority and responsibility on the governmental level or at the FDA (Food and Drug Administration of the U.S.) took serious notice of these warnings. The voices of the few who took notice were lost in a false euphoria of forthcoming solutions and optimistic predictions.

Still, nobody wants to face the facts, even today, when the world is in imminent danger not only from AIDS, but from all the degenerative diseases relentlessly on the rise. There are rumors circulating that the real numbers of AIDS victims have been changed or withheld, and that nobody is making an effort to elicit the truth. It is as if people do not want to hear that the disease is incurable, and they just pretend it doesn't exist for them until it strikes them or someone they know.

But concerned scientists who are authorities on the subject of AIDS have contrary viewpoints from the ones mentioned above, and they emphatically warn us of the dangers of the disease. Here is what they have to say:

"The following are excerpts from the testimony of Dr. John Seale before joint hearings of the California Senate Health and Human

Services Committee and Assembly Committee on Apportionment
and Elections...

- The AIDS virus is the molecular biological equivalent of the
  nuclear bomb. The genetic information contained in its tiny strip
  of RNA has all that is needed to render the human race extinct
  within 50 years...
- The optimists, like Professor Jay Levy of San Francisco, believe
  that a mere 50% will die following infection—the other 50% will
  come to little or no harm. This optimistic vision makes AIDS
  twice as deadly as smallpox, and as deadly as bubonic plague, the
  cause of the Black Death in the 14th century, which killed one-
  third of the entire population of Europe.
- The pessimists, like Professor William Haseltine of Harvard,
  believe that 100% of people infected will die within 20 years or so
  of the initial infection, as is the case with rabies virus infection.
  This is why he testified before a Senate Committee in Washington
  a year ago that AIDS was 'species-threatening.' In simple English,
  Prof. Haseltine believes the AIDS virus has the capacity to
  spread, and to kill every man, woman, and child on Earth..." [24]

I am by nature not an alarmist, and my work has always been
to save lives and bring hope to those suffering, but things have
gotten quite out of hand and I feel it is time to speak out. What
is happening on this planet at this moment is appalling. While
the situation has elicited the concern of some people, the great
majority is not only unaware of the real problem but naively
believes the statements made by established medicine.

Nobody denies that there are excellent minds battling and
struggling at this very moment to find solutions to our health
problems. The intentions are noble, the scientists honest and
dedicated, but the net result of the purely therapeutic side of
medical research is usually "hazard" rather than harmony.

Medical research, no matter how much effort, money and
dedication goes into it, always seems to give us a deceptive
answer. There are a lot of promises in the beginning which more
often than not end up in disasters. The problem is that many
times the medical drugs used to manipulate the human body are
so deep and insidious in their effects that when we finally
perceive their long-term side effects, it is usually too late; the
damage has already been done.

Today everybody thinks that it was only thalidomide and a
handful of other drugs that have been harmful, while everything
else is considered safe and "innocent." Thalidomide showed its
appalling effects upon the human organism in quite a short time
because it was a very crude drug. This was the reason why it was

soon recognized and isolated, though not without leaving some very tragic consequences in its wake. Can you imagine what could have happened if its effects had not been discovered when they were?

What we have to understand is that all chemical drugs, no matter how innocent they may appear in the beginning, are bound to have some type of effect, be it large or small, on the human organism. Some drugs or vaccinations may have such a subtle and insidious influence upon the body that their side effects may be apparent only five to ten years later.

In 1978, in my book *The Science of Homeopathy,* I advanced the theory that vaccinations deeply disturb the organism before they can protect it from a specific disease. But few have asked about the long-term effects of vaccinations. Who can really calculate the net profit or loss from such practice? We all know that vaccinations are "addressed" to the immune system and that their aim is to "force" it to produce antibodies to protect the organism from future attacks of a specific infectious disease.

This idea was really "clever," but the question still remains for future generations to answer whether it was clever enough to outsmart nature.

Several other questions which will take a long time to answer are:

- Can nature (the organism), under the stress of a vaccine, suffer an unpredictable reaction which rearranges its deeper structures of defense, such as the reticuloendothelial, immune, sympathetic and parasympathetic systems, such that it can no longer defend itself from future diseases of a different type?
- Is it possible that by using such powerful agents we are accelerating the body's manifestation of its latent predisposition for chronic diseases?
- Who can foretell, with any degree of certainty, the long-range consequences of such subtle intervention in the innermost workings of the human organism?

In my teachings, I have alluded repeatedly to the fact that we have meddled in an unwise and serious manner with the immune system, and that it is possible the present "explosion" of some of the most terrifying chronic diseases of our times—like multiple sclerosis, cancer and rheumatoid arthritis—may have been precipitated largely by certain vaccinations. Such practices may have consequences that appear ten to fifteen years after the initial vaccination, which I believe is the case with multiple sclerosis.

Is it a coincidence that underdeveloped countries which did not have obligatory vaccination programs twenty years ago have no incidence of this disease today? It is my estimation that African immigrants living in America and Europe display the same incidence of multiple sclerosis as the native populations, proving that environmental, not genetic factors are of primary etiological concern.

Arab countries in general have practically no incidence of multiple sclerosis, while Israel, whose population has migrated mostly from western countries and has had obligatory vaccinations, has one of the highest incidences of multiple sclerosis.

I do not claim that this disease has appeared only because of vaccinations, but I do believe that its alarming rate of proliferation has been accelerated by the advent of vaccinations. Vaccinations disturb the immune system, and I strongly believe that quite soon it will be established, beyond a shadow of a doubt, that multiple sclerosis is due to a specific defect in the immune system.

How responsible has the BCG vaccination (anti-tubercular) been for the "explosion" of rheumatoid arthritis in our times? In laboratory experiments on rats it has been shown beyond question that BCG vaccination creates a condition very similar to rheumatoid arthritis.

The main question that established medicine must ask is how much and **how far can we intervene** in the infinitely complex and interdependent mechanisms of the human defense system without permanently damaging its ecology?

I understand that all these ideas may sound presumptuous or arbitrary, and I also perceive that such a stand may seem like a collective rejection of all the attainments of modern medicine, but I assure you that this is definitely not my intention.

All I propose at this stage is that established medicine keep an open mind and take an intelligent, hard look at the whole health issue. At present, it does not seem to be proceeding in the right direction. Despite having achieved the appearance of protecting health and saving lives, it has not realistically estimated the cost in long-term side effects of its usual health-care practices.

If one wanted to examine the actual state of health of the western world, it would be necessary to completely halt the massive consumption of pharmaceutical drugs currently in vogue. This would be an interesting experiment, because it would allow the real picture of "health in the world" to emerge. To do this, we would have to withhold the anxiolytic, anti-psychotic, anti-epileptic drugs, all the painkillers that sedate patients, etc., and then watch the consequences.

I believe we would see terrifying scenes unfold. The violence and insanity that have been so long suppressed would erupt. We would see homicides and suicides, hear the shrieks of pain and agony, see epileptics with fits, crippled people in pain, mad people talking to ghosts, and people suffering from spasms, hysteria and fear.

Then, and only then, would we see **the world's real state of health** today. We do not know the actual number of all those who are suffering, but I don't think it is an exaggeration to say that more than half of the population of the western world is suffering from a major or minor chronic ailment and is under some kind of treatment. There are very few individuals who don't take some medication for an ailment, minor or major, within the course of a year. Can we possibly claim victory over a disease just because we manage to palliate some of its manifestations?

Let us compare the above scene with the picture of a peaceful, remote village where medical and pharmaceutical services are not available, where people treat themselves by traditional means—herbs and folk remedies. Unfortunately, there aren't many such places left in the world today. I am sure that one would not find scenes of pandemonium, as described above, in such places. The difference is not in the way of life but in the methods of treatment and prevention of diseases. Have the people of the Caucasus Mountains, who are known to live longer than anybody else on this planet, ever attributed their longevity to the "miracles" of allopathic medicine?

Established medicine must resume its work with a different mental attitude and make new efforts. It has to realize that the palliation of pain and suffering is not an adequate solution, that in fact such palliation may only create new problems or prolong existing ones.

REFERENCES:

1. JAFFE HW: National case-control study of Kaposi's sarcoma and Pneumocystis Carinii pneumonia in homosexual men: Part 1, Epidemiologic Results. *Ann Inte Med 1983; 99: 145-151*

2. MERINO HI, RICHARDS JB: An innovative program of venereal disease casefinding; treatment and education for a population of gay men. *Ann Int Med 1980; 92: 805-808*

3. LANDIS SJ: Sexually transmitted diseases among homosexuals. *Can Med Assn J 1984; 130: 370-372*

4. GUINAN ME et al: Heterosexual and homosexual patients with the Acquired Immunodeficiency Syndrome. *Ann Int Med 1984; 100: 213-218*

5. JUDSON FN: Fear of AIDS and gonorrhoea rates in homosexual men. (Letter) *Lancet, July 16, 1983; 159-160*

6. GELLAN MCA, ISON CA: Declining incidence of gonorrhoea in London: A response to fear of AIDS. (Letter) *Lancet, October 18, 1986; 920*

7. ROGERS MA: National case-control study of Kaposi's sarcoma and Pneumocystis Carinii Pneumonia in homosexual men: Part 2, Laboratory Results. *Ann Inte Med 1983; 99: 151-158*

8. PAPE JW et al: The Acquired Immunodeficiency Syndrome in Haiti. *Ann Inter Med 1985; 103: 674-678*

9. *World Health Statistics Annual 1976*

10. *World Health Statistics Annual 1981*

11. *World Health Statistics Annual 1983*

12. *World Health Statistics Annual 1985*

13. *World Health Statistics Annual 1986*

14. *Arch Neurology 1976; 33: 2-3*

15. Editorial: The prevalence and malignancy of Alzheimer's disease. *Arch Neurology 1976; 33: 217-218*

16. Diseases of the myelin sheath. *Clinical Neurology* Vol 2. Chapter 25: 19

17. *Tropical Neurology.* ed. by J. D. Spillane: 144, 169, 212-213, 246

18. BEEBE GW et al: Studies on the natural history of multiple sclerosis. *Neurology (Minneap.) 17, No. 1*

19. ALTER M, LEIBOWITZ U, SPEER J: Risk of multiple sclerosis related to age of immigration to Israel. *Arch Neuro, 1966; 15: 234*

20. DEAN G: Annual incidence, prevalence and mortality of multiple sclerosis in white South African-born and in white immigrants to South Africa. *Brit Med J 1967; 2: 724*

21. DEAN G: The multiple sclerosis problem. *Scient Amer 1970; 233, 40*

22. DEAN G, KURTZKE J: On the risk of multiple sclerosis according to age at immigration to South Africa. *Brit Med J 1971; 3: 725-729*

23. *World Health Statistics Annual 1980*

24. The AIDS virus: prognosis, transmission, and control. *EIR 1986; October 10: 65-66*

25. PAPADOPOULOS J: *Can the BCG Vaccination Cause Polyarthritis and Osteodystrophy.* (Experimental study on hamsters). Laboratory of Experimental Pharmacology. University of Athens.

Chapter 19

PRACTICAL SUGGESTIONS FOR THOSE WHO CARE TO PROTECT THEMSELVES AND OTHERS FROM AIDS

According to the many voices of concerned scientists, this planet is in imminent danger of perishing from nuclear disaster, land and water pollution, air and chemical pollution (resulting in the destruction of the ozone layer) and more. Most of these scientists are concerned about the destruction of the environment, but there is a greater danger facing the human race today—**the destruction of the "inner" ecology of the human organism**.

The AIDS syndrome is only one aspect of a much greater pattern—the relentless progression of complex chronic diseases. These diseases herald the rapid degeneration of mankind's health. Those who understand the problem have an obligation and responsibility to educate others. I feel that unless radical measures are immediately taken, we will witness consequences far more dire than those to date. Measures have to be taken on various levels:

1. Individual level
2. Family level
3. Societal level
4. National Governmental level
5. International level

We shall enumerate some measures that pertain mostly to those concerned with AIDS, but nevertheless, similar ideas may be applied to the whole problem of degeneration of the human organism. The following thoughts, given in the form of suggestions and questions, do not cover the subject wholly but are indicative of the basic thoughts I feel are pertinent at the moment.

On the Individual level

I have divided the whole population into three groups:

1. Those who have manifested the disease in its full form.
2. Those who have the AIDS-related complex.
3. Those who do not have the disease.

We shall examine these groups separately since the "psychology" of each group differs drastically from the others.

1. Those who already have the disease:
a. What they can do for themselves
The idea here is to strengthen the immune system as much as possible by any means available and at the same time avoid anything that disturbs or damages the immune system.

Improved diets consisting of natural healthy foods, spending time in the outdoors, exercise programs, and the application of natural therapies like Homeopathy*, which by their very nature strengthen the body's defenses, are definitely indicated. I do not mean to suggest that these are the final measures of curing the disease, yet it is possible that they can improve the organism's general state of health and postpone considerably the final outcome.

A positive attitude and the determination to abandon unhealthy practices, especially those propagating recurrences of venereal infections, is not only helpful but essential.

I feel a note of warning is especially due those who decide to turn to alternative therapies. The field is full of incompetent, unscrupulous people who try to exploit this dangerous situation. The prospective patient should investigate all references before choosing a Homeopath and should always look for someone trained in classical Homeopathy, be it a medical doctor or another health practitioner. One of the indications of a good Homeopath is that he gives but one remedy at a time, observes the results and acts accordingly (see appendix).

---

* Samuel Hahnemann and the Law of Similars

"The physician's highest and only calling is to restore health to the sick, which is called Healing."

—Samuel Hahnemann
Excerpts from the author's book: *Homeopathy: Medicine of the New Man.*[7]

Homeopathy is a very highly systematic method of powerfully stimulating the body's vital force to cure illness. It is based on a few simple but profoundly insightful truths of Nature which are contrary to commonly held beliefs.

In all its ramifications, homeopathy is far too sophisticated a discipline to be learned in a few seminars or by reading this book. The principles are simple in concept, but difficult to fully comprehend, and they require years of intensive training and experience to apply—as many, and more, years as are required in a standard medical school.

To properly introduce homeopathy, we must go back 170 years and examine perhaps the most remarkable story in medical history, entirely encompassed in the life of one man.

With time, I am certain that this man will rank as one of the greatest in medical history, alongside such giants of discovery as Einstein, Newton, and Hippocrates. Like these men, his insights have radically and permanently altered our perceptions of not only health and disease, but also the nature of existence itself. For this reason, we shall trace the life and thought of this man in some detail as a means of explaining and clarifying the basic principles of homeopathy.

In 1810, a book entitled *Organon of the Art of Healing* was published in Torgau, a small town in Germany. Its author, Samuel Hahnemann, was an extremely prominent physician and medical author of the time, so that the appearance of another book under his name generated automatic interest. However, once the book was read, the European medical community was thrown into an uproar, for Hahnemann had introduced an entirely new and radical system of medicine, one fundamentally opposed to the traditional medicine of its time.

Hahnemann called his new medicine homeopathy, a word taken from the Greek *omoeos*, meaning 'similar', and *pathos*, meaning 'suffering'. Thus, homeopathy means 'to treat with something that produces an effect similar to the suffering'. In his book, Hahnemann laid out the laws and principles of the science, gathered empirically over a period of twenty years.

Briefly, Hahnemann showed that:

1. A medical cure is brought about in accordance with certain laws of healing that exist in nature.
2. Nobody can cure outside these laws.
3. There are no diseases as such, but only diseased individuals.
4. An illness is always dynamic by nature, so the remedy must also be in a dynamic state if it is to cure.
5. The patient needs only one particular remedy and no other at any stage of his illness. Unless that certain remedy is found, his condition will not be cured but, at best, be only temporarily relieved.

Because of its dramatically curative results, homeopathy was soon to win widespread approval throughout Europe and the world, but when Hahnemann's work was first published, it met with the most bitter opposition from doctors still prescribing blood-letting, cathartics, and diaphoretics. Hahnemann was not discouraged. He was a brilliant individual and, as such, was accustomed to being misunderstood.

His first biographer, Thomas Bradford, describes how Hahnemann's father used to lock his son up with what he called 'thinking exercises' —problems the boy was required to solve himself. In this way Hahnemann learned to develop the use of intuition and insight, and to come to know the limitations of intellectual logic.

Clearly, Hahnemann was precocious at virtually everything he attempted. When he was twelve, his teacher had him teaching Greek to the other students. He put himself through university studies of chemistry and medicine by translating English books into German. He qualified as a physician from the University of Leipzig in 1779, and soon after began publishing a series of works on medicine and chemistry. In 1791, his research in chemistry earned him election to the Academy of Science in Mayence. His *Apothecary's Lexicon* became a standard textbook of the time, and he was chosen from all the physicians in Germany to standardize the German *Pharmacopoeia*.

Hahnemann dropped the practice of medicine, much to the dismay of his colleagues and friends. As he wrote to one friend:

"It was agony for me to walk always in the darkness, when I had to heal the sick and to prescribe, according to such or such an hypothesis concerning diseases, substances which owed their place in the *Materia Medica* to an arbitrary decision...Soon after my marriage, I renounced the practice of medicine, that I might no longer incur the risk of doing injury, and I engaged exclusively in chemistry, and in literary occupations."

He could have made a very comfortable living practicing medicine, but he preferred poverty to the necessity of conforming to a system 'whose errors and uncertainties disgusted (him).'

Hahnemann's active mind nevertheless remained curious, open and systematic. He relentlessly probed into the basic issues of health and disease. It was in this frame of mind that he stumbled onto the first fundamental principle of homeopathy. He was translating the *Materia Medica* written by Professor Cullen of London University. Cullen devoted twenty pages of this book to the therapeutic indication of Peruvian Bark (a source of what is known today as quinine), attributing its success in the treatment of malarias to the fact that it was bitter. Hahnemann was so dissatisfied with this explanation that he did something very extraordinary: he took a series of doses of Peruvian Bark himself! This was an action entirely unprecedented in the medical world of his time. It is not known to this day what prompted him to do such a thing, but his experiment led to an entirely new era of medicine. He describes the result as follows:

"I took by way of experiment, twice a day, four drachms of good China (Peruvian Bark). My feet, finger ends, etc., at first became cold; I grew languid and drowsy; then my heart began to palpitate, and my pulse grew hard and small; intolerable anxiety, trembling, prostration throughout all my limbs; then pulsation in my head, redness of my cheeks, thirst, and in short, all the symptoms, which are ordinarily characteristic of intermittent fever made their appearance one after the other, yet without the peculiar chilly, shivering rigor.

Briefly, even those symptoms which are of regular occurrence and especially characteristic—as the stupidity of mind, the kind of rigidity in all the limbs, but above all the numb, disagreeable sensation which seems to have its seat in the periosteum, over every bone in the body—all these made their appearance. This paroxysm lasted two or three hours each time and recurred if I repeated this dose, not otherwise; I discontinued it, and was in good health."

Imagine the astounding revelation that struck Hahnemann as a result of his experiment! The standard medical assumption had always been that if the body produces a symptom, a medicine must be given to relieve that symptom. This was so deeply ingrained that it had almost become an automatic reflex in the mind of doctor and patient. But here, in his own personal experience, Hahnemann found that a drug which was known to be curative in malaria actually produces those very symptoms when given to a healthy person.

Many would simply have ignored such an observation as a mere exception. Hahnemann, however, was a true empirical scientist. To him, the observation itself was what counted—regardless of whether it fitted neatly into current dogmas or not. He accepted the observation and went on to make further experiments which further proved this 'chance' observation as a fact of Nature: *A substance which produces symptoms in a healthy person cures those symptoms in a sick person.*

Hahnemann and his colleagues recognized in these symptom pictures the identical symptomatologies of many people seeking cures. These medicines were then tried on patients who manifested similar symptoms, and the amazing discovery was made that the drugs actually cured so-called "incurable" diseases when prescribed according to this principle. According to the law he had discovered, Hahnemann saw that every drug must necessarily cure the set of symptoms it produces in a healthy human organism.

The process by which Hahnemann and his colleagues experimentally produced the symptoms of a substance upon their healthy organisms he called "proving". Orthodox medicine (which homeopaths term "allopathic", from *allo,* meaning "other") also has its process of proving drugs, but with the very important difference that it experiments upon animals.

Animals do not possess the power of speech. They cannot report the subtleties of alterations in mood or the different types of pain which can be described by human experimental subjects. In addition, the physiology of animals is considerably different from that of the human being. Hahnemann perceived clearly that any therapeutic system based upon animal experimentation must be done within the same realms of physiology and awareness as the medicines will be called upon to act therapeutically. This principle is merely common sense, yet it was absolutely revolutionary in Hahnemann's time.

Hahnemann's rationale for the homeopathic principle, known today as the Law of Similars, is explained in Aphorism 19 of the *Organon:*

"Now the diseases are nothing more than alterations in the state of health of the healthy individual which express themselves by morbid (i.e., disease-producing) signs, and the cure is also only possible by a change to the healthy condition from the state of health of the diseased individual; it is very evident that medicines could never cure diseases if they did not possess the power of altering man's state of health which depends upon sensations and functions: indeed, that their curative power must be owing solely to this power they possess of altering man's state of health."

Preparation of Homeopathic remedies

Once Hahnemann felt he had proven enough remedies, he began prescribing them in the accepted dosages of the time; but although the patient was invariably cured, the drug often caused such a severe initial aggravation of symptoms that patients and doctors alike became alarmed. Such aggravation was to be expected since the drug itself was producing symptoms similar to those of the patient. Hahnemann wanted to test some of the drugs in common use at that time—drugs such as mercury and arsenic; but, of course, he could not give such toxic substances to healthy people.

So he reduced the dose to one-tenth of its customary amount. The patient was still cured but the aggravation though lighter, remained. Hahnemann diluted the remedy still further, each time prescribing only one-tenth of the previous dose, and presently reached a dilution that had essentially no more medicine left in it.

Precisely at this most critical juncture, Hahnemann made another amazing discovery. To this day, it is not exactly known how Hahnemann came upon the procedure. In any case, he simply submitted each dilution to a series of vigorous shakes (or "succussions" as he called them) and discovered that progressive dilutions became not only less toxic but also more potent!

Hahnemann had found a solution to the problem that had occupied medical men throughout history. He had beaten the problem of the "side effects" of drugs!

Hahnemann says that the efficacy of a remedy thus processed is increased because "the powers, which are, as it were, hidden and dormant in the crude drug, are developed and roused into activity to an incredible degree."

Hahnemann first considered that distilled water, alcohol, and lactose were medicinally inert, so he diluted the medicines in these substances. If the remedy was diluted in water or alcohol, he mixed one part of the substance with ninety-nine parts of the liquid and submitted the mixture to one hundred vigorous succussions. This dynamized solution he called the "first centesimal potency". Then he mixed one part of this first potency with ninety-nine parts of water or alcohol and again succussed the dilution one hundred times to produce the second centesimal potency. The third step in the process, of course, diluted the initial substance to one part in a million, the fourth step to one part in a hundred million, and so on. He repeated it up to thirty times and

apparently did not go beyond that himself, although modern homeopaths use potencies to the hundred-thousandth centesimal and beyond!

The implications of this discovery are staggering. A substance
shaken and diluted to a dilution of 1 in 100,000 parts, even to a total of
60 zeros and more, still acts to cure disease, quickly and permanently,
and without side effects!

Clearly this phenomenon cannot be explained by ordinary chemical
mechanisms. The dilutions are so astronomical that not even a molecule of the original medicines is left! And yet the actual clinical results
demonstrate beyond a doubt that some influence remains—an influence which is powerful enough to cure even deep chronic diseases. In
aphorism 209, Hahnemann writes:

> "The homeopathic system of medicine develops, because of its
> special use, to a hitherto unheard of degree, the inner medicinal
> powers of the crude substances by means of a process peculiar to it,
> hitherto never tried, whereby they become immeasurably and pen-
> etratingly efficacious and remedial."

What Hahnemann has discovered is that there lies hidden in every
substance in Nature some inner life. We can mobilize and use this
"force" if we know how to process the substance correctly.

Somehow, the repeated dilutions and succussions of a homeopathic
medicine release a great curative energy which is inherent in the
substance. In homeopathy we witness the amazing cures that the
potentized remedy can bring about.

In this connection, we are struck by something which the famed
healer Paracelsus wrote centuries ago:

> "The Quintessence is that which is extracted from a
> substance...After it has been cleansed of all impurities and its
> perishable parts, and refined to the highest degree, it attains
> extraordinary powers and perfections...In it there is great purity,
> and that has the virtue to cleanse the body."

As we have seen in the holistic health field—not to mention the ideas
of Einstein and modern quantum physics—we have gone beyond the
concept of nineteenth-century materialism and accepted quite easily
the idea that all matter is in fact energy, and that this energy can be
released and even harnessed. The true miracle is that in homeopathy
it has been harnessed for the cure of the disease.

---

b. What they can do for others

The first obligation that everyone with AIDS has is a moral
one, and that is to restrict sexual contact with others because of
the grave possibility of infecting them.

Those who have understood the general principles involved in
this book should attempt to educate others and to impress upon

them the necessity of not becoming involved in situations where
the risk of venereal infection is great.

Those who are suspected of having the disease should by their
own volition go to AIDS testing centers where their identities
would be kept in confidence. The decision to reveal to others
whether or not one is a carrier is left up to the integrity of the
individual.

Every one of us is responsible for the state in which humanity
finds itself at the moment, and it is quite unfair to start
"throwing stones" and blaming others for what lies squarely
with us and our conscience.

I believe the great majority of the victims are responsible
people who understand the implications and the potential
tensions to which this issue can give rise.

2. Those who have the AIDS-related complex:

This group has a much better chance of survival than the first
group. The patients should immediately start a program of
"rejuvenating" their immune system by turning to good alternative therapies, especially Homeopathy and other auxiliary measures, already mentioned above. Although at the moment there
isn't enough evidence that good Homeopathic treatment can
really cure such individuals, there is a good chance of improving
their plight.

It is imperative for them not to stress their immune systems
any further by taking drugs, illicit or otherwise, and to be careful
in their sexual practices so they won't be infected with new
venereal diseases. Here the idea of the vulnerability of the
immune system, which is already under stress, and the damage
that would be done to it under new and repeated attacks of
venereal disease, cannot be emphasized enough.

3. Those who do not have the disease:

This is, of course, the major part of the population. These
persons should be the most responsible for keeping up their own
health as well as the health of others. I would strongly suggest
to these people that they turn to alternative methods when
treatment is needed, especially to Homeopathy. Even if they
have to resort to allopathic drugs for a short period of time, they
should then abstain from further drug-taking so that their
immune systems can recuperate. Most of all, they should try to

keep from contracting venereal disease, which would again require treatment with antibiotics. The main dictum should be to maintain the integrity of the immune system by disturbing it as little as possible and supporting it as much as possible by intelligent measures. A good diet and moderate exercise are always necessary and important in maintaining a healthy lifestyle, but keeping away from strong drugs is even more important.

Even though the majority of the allopathic profession today denies or ignores alternative methods of therapy such as Homeopathy, Acupuncture, Osteopathy and Naturopathy, and even though we may not have conclusive proof now that these alternative therapies work to the extent that their exponents claim, people should at least try to find out for themselves about the merits, the pros and cons, of such treatments. And here I speak mostly about Homeopathy since I have been an eyewitness to its positive results for the past 30 years. The fact that these methods do not cause serious side effects makes the argument for their use even stronger.

Here I must stress again the necessity of finding a good classical Homeopath who will prescribe only one remedy at a time, observe the results, and not mix the remedies by practicing "polypharmacy." The difference between classical Homeopathy and Homeopathic polypharmacy is indeed enormous, and people should not confuse one with the other.

On the Family level

a. Protecting the family member that has AIDS:
It is an absolute certainty that the family of the AIDS victim faces many difficult problems and will be called to answer questions that they probably had never before imagined. The main dilemma will be that of cohabitation; how will parents face jeopardizing the lives of their other children, threatening them with potential death. They must ask themselves what kind of attention they should give to the diseased ones and to what extent they should allow contact among themselves.

Again, the answers here cannot be cut and dried, and there will be a lot of different responses depending on the closeness of the family. If love prevails, it will be much easier to see the answers and to make the necessary adjustments.

b. The responsibility of the family towards society

Life will nevertheless be a constant stress under these circumstances. The family members will have to undergo frequent checkups and report immediately to health authorities the infection of another member of the family and the exact circumstances under which it took place. Health authorities should be informed as soon as possible since this information could be invaluable to other families in the same situation.

At this stage I will not go as far as others and proclaim that the species is in danger of vanishing within twenty to fifty years, but I am very aware of the fact that human organisms are developing degenerative diseases which definitely will be species-endangering in the very near future.

A good sign at this moment is that people are afraid of AIDS and have what might be called an "AIDS Scare Syndrome" which is so great that it has reduced casual sexual contact enormously. As a result of this trend, we shall witness a decrease in the number of sexually transmitted diseases, and as a secondary effect of this reduction, the number of AIDS cases may eventually decrease. In any case, such a decline will not be apparent for a long time since many, perhaps millions, who have been subclinically harboring the AIDS virus will become symptomatic in the foreseeable future.

AIDS, like cancer and many other chronic, degenerative diseases, has posed insoluble questions to the medical profession. My point of view is that if we cannot solve any of these problems, the least we can do is to stop and think for a moment about the **possible reasons which may have led us to such dead ends**. Pretending the problem does not exist is not a solution that will carry us far.

On the Societal level

Society faces a major dilemma since AIDS is not only an infectious disease but one that is lethal as well. The first of society's reactions would be to ostracize the AIDS victims in order to save itself. This attitude is certainly not going to work because AIDS is not a disease of homosexuals, as I have tried to show throughout this book, **but a disease of our society which evolved as a result of more complex conditions.** It has come about because of the greed, irresponsibility, indifference, competition and so on that society has not only allowed but promoted.

The average person cannot imagine the pharmaceutical companies' wealth and power, growing ever more with each new turn of profit. They tell us that the billions of dollars in profit are in return given back to society through research. When has a pharmaceutical company ever given money for promoting research that was outside its own narrow interests? When has their research ever proven to be of any lasting value? The above rationale, justifying their profits, is only an excuse; the facts are that these companies use profits for power and control.

Medical history has shown us that there has been a long series of discoveries of new drugs which were first presented as "wonders" and "miracle drugs" and soon proved to have devastatingly harmful side effects. The scenario has become almost stereotypical. A drug is first promoted as a breakthrough in scientific research; a certain time period elapses where its real side effects became apparent; and not long after that it is proclaimed a menace to health, a carcinogen, an extremely hazardous drug.

Was there ever any substantial amount of money given by any large pharmaceutical company to promote research on **alternative therapeutic systems**?

The public should read such books as Milton Silverman's *Pills, Profits and Politics,* Ivan Illich's *Medical Nemesis,* Martin's *Hazards of Medication,* and Braithwaite's *Corporate Crime in the Pharmaceutical Industry.*

Greed and irresponsibility have not only affected the pharmaceutical companies and their directors or promoters, but society as a whole at every level, whether related to medicine or not.

We are using the pharmaceutical industry and its invisible "branches" as a paradigm because of the main theme of this book, but I feel that every one of us must bear a share of the responsibility for the deterioration of our society as a whole.

The way pharmaceutical companies promote and market a drug is irresponsible, but who can claim that he has never been irresponsible in the basic issues of life, such as raising children, reacting to a dispute with a neighbor over property, dealing with a job, etc. Society cannot put the blame on pharmaceutical companies or homosexuals or promiscuity *per se,* because all are products of our way of life.

For instance, who can say with any degree of certainty that the same homosexuality does not stem from the effects on mothers' hormonal systems induced by the standard practice of feeding livestock and dairy cows various hormones and antibiotics to facilitate growth and production?

The mere possibility that such thoughts may be valid should make us all pause and think of our own responsibilities as members of the societies in which we live. Many of us know better, but out of laziness or apathy or other various reasons, we let such practices continue unopposed. Very few have taken the initiative to inform society of its peril, and now we find ourselves confronted by the spectre of AIDS.

Organized societies have to come up with the right answers. People should not rest on their laurels and think that it is none of their business, that such epidemics will not affect them. It is up to society to decide the best way to handle the issue, and many hard decisions lie ahead.

On the National Governmental level

On the national level, immediate measures have to be taken by the responsible agencies to uncover the real causes of the recurring medical catastrophes that have plagued western civilization for the last few decades.

These agencies have to realize that those endangered are not the "simple" or primitive societies, but rather those who live in the very heart of technological civilization.

We try to reason the cause of disease by giving answers such as "the extreme stress under which we live" or the "pollution of the atmosphere". These are not precise enough explanations to have any significant meaning with regard to the management of diseases or the prevention of the deterioration of health of whole populations in these countries. One may also argue that the parameters involved in this degeneration are too numerous and complex to be isolated. This is true to an extent, but the argument of this book remains that the probable **main cause** of this deterioration is the chemical drugging that has prevailed over the last thirty years.

If governments are not prepared to take aggressive action, to look for immediate solutions to our health dilemma, my feeling is that our continued survival is in doubt.

People in government have to realize that they and their families are not exempt from the snowballing processes which culminate in epidemics and chronic diseases; it is time they showed concern and sensitivity towards such vital and delicate matters.

The public in general should put pressure on these agencies to keep an open mind on issues of health and make them listen to responsible voices that raise concerns and propose solutions.

I do not claim to be the most articulate or authoritative advocate of this cause; many other people are also voicing their concern, but yet to no avail.

What we are saying is that in spite of the fact that it is already very late, nobody seems ready to take any initiative. The public perhaps expects everything to be initiated by the government, while the government, because of its structure and inertia, moves slowly and laboriously, probably expecting the public to put pressure on it first before initiating any new "radical" action. As a result, we witness a fatalistic attitude from both the government and the public, each one claiming that they have done "their best" and there is nothing more to be done. The truth of the matter is that what has been done to date has been highly inadequate.

The most important function of government, at least at this moment, is to connect those people who are aware of the ongoing destruction of this planet with the responsible agencies which have access to the information, authority and financial means needed to institute new, creative ideas which might reverse our destructive spiral.

It appears that our societies are extremely inflexible in structure, such that only a really big "shock" can shake us free and bring about an essential change. This "shock" has already occurred, and its unembellished dimensions are sufficient cause for initiating change.

Another one of government's duties is to start a real investigation of alternative therapies such as Homeopathy, Acupuncture, Osteopathy, Herbalism and Naturopathy—all employing less toxic means for combating diseases.

Objective trials should show the relative suitability of such therapies, and then the government could organize and encourage their extensive use. Certainly the resulting broad range of clinical experience will help these therapeutic disciplines further realize their potential and further enhance and refine their methods.

On the International level

On this level the role and importance of the World Health Organization (WHO) is paramount.

Its officials should be the first ones acquainted with the real facts emerging from statistical analysis and global collection of information. The statisticians should be able to study the facts correctly, and a "think-tank" should be employed to interpret general trends in health care, to evaluate different kinds of therapeutic disciplines and finally to advise the different governmental agencies.

This *Model* suggests, for instance, that the average lifespan within western societies will soon start showing a downward trend due to constant epidemics, new acute diseases and the explosion of chronic incurable diseases. Soon the statistics will have to take into consideration the **quality of life** and find ways to measure it. It is for this reason that WHO will have to define health and disease more precisely, so that the statistics can have a point of reference. The present definition of health accepted by WHO is insufficient and overlooks a number of important factors. A symposium on the "Definition of Health" should be organized by international agencies like WHO.

The *Model* also suggests that the **quality** of life has already dropped dramatically. The increase of anxiety, insecurity and chronic diseases in general have compromised that quality despite the advancements in technology over the last twenty years which were supposed to ease working conditions and improve life.

The *Model* also suggests that the way in which we have tried to fight disease has so far been flawed; the results have been misleading and, in the long run, devastating. The *Model* tries to point out that the "quick-fix" methods used in curing "non-serious" ailments have driven them deeper into the recesses of the organism and thus created more severe diseases. If this statement holds true, then we must painfully acknowledge that the whole civilized world is on a course toward self-destruction.

We may be destroying the human race under the pretense of saving it. One wonders why it is that man has been so deluded about so vital an issue as health. One disconcerting possibility is that such calamities as have been recounted on these pages are the inescapable consequence of our societies' way of life.

The diminution of AIDS will not come soon, and if it comes at all, it will only be after drastic changes have taken place.

I understand this all sounds a bit too pessimistic to be true. We all tend to think that since we have survived for so long, our continued existence as a species is assured despite such catastrophic epidemics as AIDS. However, I sincerely believe that without drastic alterations of our prevailing methods of health care, the quality of our survival, itself in doubt, will be severely compromised.

REFERENCES:

1. HAHNEMANN S: *The Organon of the Art of Healing*. Economic Homeo Stores Private Ltd., 1921. B Jain New Delhi reprint
2. HAHNEMANN S: *Chronic Diseases*. Economic Homeo Stores Private Ltd. B Jain New Delhi reprint
3. HAHNEMANN S: *Materia Medica Pura*. Economic Homeo Stores Private Ltd. B Jain New Delhi reprint
4. BRADFORD TL: *Life and Letters of Dr. Samuel Hahnemann*. Philadelphia: Boericke and Tafel, 1895
5. KENT JT: *Lectures on Homeopathic Philosophy*. Berkeley: North Atlantic Books, 1980
6. KENT JT: *Lectures on Homeopathic Materia Medica*. Calcutta, India: Jain Publishers Co.
7. VITHOULKAS G: *Homeopathy, Medicine of the New Man*. New York: ARCO Publishing, Inc., 1979

EPILOGUE

Some pertinent theoretical questions:

—Why have we allowed ourselves to arrive at this state of affairs?

—What deeper reasons were involved in humanity's following an impotent therapeutic system that involved so much suffering and pain?

—Is the AIDS syndrome an unavoidable projection of existing degeneration occurring in our everyday life?

—Why is it almost impossible to see what is right and true, and why do we usually follow what is wrong and elusive?

—Why is it mankind's fate to accuse and crucify its pioneers while at the same time glorifying the demagogue, the superficial and the hypocrite?

—Why do the masses always follow what is mediocre and materialistic, unable to perceive subtler but truer realities?

—Is it reasonable to expect inner peace and serenity when we ourselves promote competition and aggression in the "outside" world?

—Is it conceivable that these questions can be answered by a society which promotes injustice and tolerates crime in all its intricate forms?

—Can we demand to live without pain and suffering when greed and selfishness have been "cherished" human qualities for so long?

—Doesn't everybody know that these qualities bring along with them pain and suffering?

These are some of the basic questions we are called upon to answer during moments of crisis when our demands for relief from suffering rise excruciatingly high.

One could say that suffering is manifested in our societies because of the very values we project and will only end if we change these values. I do not exclude anyone from such accusations, including myself. I have known in my life highly evolved spiritual individuals who were also not entirely free from the more subtle forms of greed and selfishness.

—Is it then perhaps logical to think that such a society deserves the kind of medical treatment it has thus far received ?

—Is it possible that the medical establishment thinks itself exempt from fallacy?

—Is the medical establishment's aggressiveness and competitive behavior only a representation of the behavior long present in our society?

—Is it possible that at a certain point in time the idealism (thoughts to save humanity, etc.) amongst medical students is replaced by the more materialistic conviction that studying medicine is the best financial investment?

I fully expect responses to these questions will vary, and I believe that they can be truly answered only when each physician individually confronts his conscience. Unfortunately, we cannot ask "systems" to face their consciences. It is individuals who are responsible for our various "systems." There is an anonymity and vagueness to organized health systems behind which the individual employee can hide. The individual's conscience is somewhat protected by such systems, and his feelings of guilt are allayed by the fact that he does not feel personally responsible for what is taking place. One can accuse the medical establishment and its affiliated organizations *ad infinitum,* but I am neither a moralist nor a fatalist. I have always believed in **doing** something to improve ourselves and the societies in which we live, though such changes have almost invariably come after much suffering and great calamities. I suppose what I am looking for is the best action to take under the present circumstances.

I have no delusions, and I do not expect the ideas contained in this treatise to be readily accepted by the medical establishment. On the contrary, I am certain that even if there is a widespread, general acceptance by the scientific community, there will always be members of the medical establishment who will find excuses and different reasons for continuing the status quo.

The deeper reasons for this state of affairs:

I believe the major contributing factor to the appalling situation in which we find ourselves is the fact that the medical establishment **monopolized the right to provide medical services** and created a very rigid and conservative system. It seems that even if a therapeutic miracle were to take place and it were outside this system, it would, in the name of science, only be criticized or condemned as quackery.

Established medicine has remained without a rival, without constructive criticism, and finally without "heart" for far too long.

Whenever a member of the medical society has tried to criticize the system from within, he or she has been ostracized or threatened with the revocation of his/her medical license; at the least, their professional standing has suffered *(Confessions of a Medical Heretic*: Mendelson*)*. The hold which medical associations have on their members is formidable. Many of the medical community's most sensitive and perceptive members have at times felt a sense of suffocation and despair at the hands of these associations.

If one observes history, one can see that as societies became more and more organized and civilized, medical systems took over and monopolized the "health" situation. Their initial goal was the protection of the health of the people, but this initial goal eventually yielded to the desire for material wealth and gain. This observation is aptly put forth in the book *Pills, Profits and Politics: The Corporate Crime of the Pharmaceutical Industry.*

But as countries progressed and became technologically more advanced, more and more health problems came to the forefront. In such countries as Sweden, Norway, Denmark, England and Holland alternative methods of therapy could be freely applied by people who were not medical doctors. The medical establishments of some of these countries repeatedly tried to force their governments to take action against such lay practitioners, but to no avail. In fact their efforts brought about a diametrically opposite effect; many more flocked to alternative therapies.

In this way a "free market" was created in which only the reputation and results of the practitioner mattered, not his or her credentials. It is true that because of this freedom, some health practitioners emerged who took advantage of the relatively unstructured order of things in the beginning, when alternative therapies were just coming into their own.

In the meantime, several members of the medical community joined the ranks of those practicing alternative medicine. Most of these physicians joined the alternative movement because their experience with established medicine had made them aware of the fallacies inherent in that system. These were the medical doctors, according to my estimation, who had not lost their primary goal in entering the medical field, these were the people who were most sensitive to human suffering. They understood and perceived the confusion, despair and futility that plagued medical orthodoxy. These medical doctors, more often than not, felt isolated from mainstream medicine because, unlike their colleagues, they questioned the existing medical practices. They were in a very difficult situation, as they came into conflict with many of the classical doctrines taught in medical colleges. The questions they raised remained unanswered for quite a long time because of reprisals from the medical community; but as a seed takes root, so did the questions and discontent about official treatments evolve within the medical ranks. Established medicine chose to ignore these questions put forth by many of its most illustrious members and proceeded, oblivious to the conflict within its own ranks. About this time, many people as well as the media sensed the truth of the matter and supported the alternative movement. But there were no organized medical centers of alternative therapies with enough prestige to replace the existing institutions, apart from some heroic attempts by the Naturopathic Schools in the U.S.

The need for expanding alternative methods of therapy:

Therefore, the only hope left is to create **new medical centers** to fill the majority of today's therapeutic demands. The old "arteriosclerotic" systems will eventually sink into oblivion, abandoned by a public which on the one hand will have become aware of the hazards of allopathic medicine, and on the other hand will have discovered the new possibilities offered by alternative therapies. Such methods have already proven to be more humane and quite effective when properly applied.

It stands to reason that alternative methods of therapy would have disappeared a long time ago if it were not for the real benefit they offer. I am sure that if we could have a world survey of how many people were really benefited by alternative therapeutic methods and how many were harmed by present medical therapies, the numbers in favor of alternatives would be very impressive indeed. Even the most hard-core supporter of allopathic medicine could not help but be impressed with these results. A revolution in medicine is not unthinkable at this time, but it would best be accomplished as a mild and subtle transformation rather than an abrupt or aggressive change.

In order that a peaceful revolution-transformation of such dimension can come to fruition, the "alternative school" should evolve to a point where it really deserves its new position. In order to reach this "deserving" state, existing standards have to be raised tremendously. But as soon as we bring into the picture the issue of the raising of standards, we are introducing the spectre of control. Automatically we raise the possibility of a monopoly once again, which as we have mentioned already, was the reason for the downfall of allopathic medicine.

There should not be another artificial system created with the same "arteriosclerotic" problems as those of established medicine. New schools should develop naturally by reason of necessity and worthiness, and they should contain within themselves the "seed of dissolution" in case they change too drastically for the worse.

I do not intend to relate in this book all my thoughts concerning these complex problems because I believe it to be a Herculean task, one which needs other enlightened minds to come together in a symposium under the auspices of global organizations. They could start by discussing the need for such schools and setting certain standards for their establishment. I would like to offer some initial thoughts on the subject.

I foresee that in the near future the field of therapeutics will be the main battleground for almost all sciences, since the demand for better health services will be so acute that much human effort will be concentrated in these areas. Therefore, it is bound to attract many competent scientists and warrant competition as well. The quest for effective knowledge will be so great that competition in this field will be formidable.

I would therefore propose a drastic change in the policies of governments and health agencies. Instead of subsidizing the patient by paying his cost for receiving "harmful" treatment,

they should subsidize health practitioners to gain the appropriate knowledge and only partly subsidize the patient. The reason is that health practitioners are the main advocates and seekers of the best therapeutic knowledge and are eyewitness to the systems which really benefit patients; thus, they in their turn are qualified to seek out the best possible schools and teachers because they and their patients will both benefit from this knowledge. Governments and insurance companies should pool their efforts in producing good and efficient health practitioners, rather than paying the huge costs of medical treatment which more often than not create more sickness than health. At the present time, governments and responsible agencies alike are caught in a vicious cycle because of tremendous costs and unforeseen future consequences for the health of the general public. A worldwide informational campaign should be started so people have the facts about allopathic medicine and its consequences. This will help relieve them of their naive notions of the well-advertised "miracle drugs" and will help them to think for themselves and judge accordingly.

In my estimation, another concept which has destroyed allopathic medicine is the idea that an institution, a medical school, can give **exclusive right** to practice medicine without teaching the students the necessary lessons of "humanism."

I say this because the factors such as ability, intention, sacrifice and compassion needed to be a healer have been completely ignored. The main priority taken into consideration is whether the student has answered certain technical questions correctly in the examination. Afterwards, the state medical licensing agency enters the picture and bestows the lucky individual with the "license to practice medicine"— in other words, with the exclusive, unconditional right to deal with people's health. But that is not all; they also manage to pass laws which punish anyone practicing an alternative method of therapy and who do not belong to their associations.

It has also been silently agreed that medical doctors will give account of their actions only to the medical association to which they belong.

I believe it is difficult for people outside the medical establishment to realize the intricacies and the extreme control inherent in such situations. Finally, because of the relegation of the patient to so "unfair" and subordinate a position, the idea of malpractice emerged in the United States, and with it another very profitable "business racket" was born.

Many times patients sue for the slightest cause, and insurance premiums for physicians as well as patients have risen accordingly. The final outcome has been that the American patient is paying a lot of money for medical services which he can get elsewhere in the world, such as Europe, at a much lower price.

Physicians have become increasingly concerned, not only about the welfare of the patient, but also about protecting themselves against a lawsuit. So in order to safeguard their position and not fall prey to any malpractice suits, they "over-prescribe." What this means is that although the physician knows, for instance, that the patient is a terminal cancer case, he will prescribe chemotherapy anyway, or prescribe antibiotics for a case which does not warrant them.

Such situations are leading some physicians to seek alternative solutions and to abandon a system so rigidly constructed that it leaves little if any room for change. Some, out of despair or ignorance of an alternative route to better therapies and health, have chosen to sacrifice their very expensive education and years of study and opt for other professions that weigh less on their conscience.

There are a lot of other reasons why this exclusivity the medical profession has secured for itself does not benefit either the patient or the profession. There is only one way that governmental agencies can correct the situation: Promote alternative methods of therapy so that allopathic medicine will have a worthy rival.

The New Centers of Medical Education

I envision schools that will be centers of real knowledge, which will provide an education far exceeding the technical and strictly "medical" aspect. Teachers from different sciences will be invited to impart their knowledge on different health issues and raise important questions for the advancement of the science. Philosophers will come to discuss the meaning of life and death in an intellectually stimulating environment, provoking students to learn and think more profoundly. Sociologists will come to share views on future societies and the improvements which should take place. Artists should come to the schools to give students a feeling for art. Ecology will be another important aspect of the educational programs. But most of all, the school will need spiritual mentors who have perceived another dimension to life and can impart to the students their wisdom and teachings of love and compassion—all necessary to the whole human being. In short, these schools will prepare students to become true healers and pillars of society.

All these special teachers will not only provide the necessary knowledge for treating disease but will shape the moral foundations of students in the best possible way, preparing them to become the initiates of a "New Society" which will attempt to provide more justice and happiness. Today the world urgently needs such educational centers, and I am sure it has the resources to build them.

What is extremely important at this moment is that knowledge be made available that can really benefit the patient and society. Much of this information has not been advanced as it should have; instead it has been suppressed.

Students from these new schools should receive this broad education over a period of at least eight years, so that before they start practicing they will have enough experience of life. Their education should be free of charge.

I would also expect that the students who graduate from such centers will get a "degree" but not a **"license"** to practice medicine. The school should give only knowledge, not privileges. The privileges will be earned in the application of their science in everyday practice, where their understanding and knowledge will be tested constantly.

Another issue which has to be discussed at length is the selection process of the students. The people who organize these schools should take care to choose the right students. The idea of "selection" should continue until the last day of their education, and only the most able and dedicated should be allowed to graduate. It is for this reason that the students' education should be supported by government and insurance agency funds, and not by the students themselves. To be accepted to such a school would be considered a great distinction, automatically drawing the admiration, respect and support of society.

It is my belief that only such graduates will be able to correctly treat a patient and take into consideration the familial and social factors which might have led this particular individual to a diseased state. The graduate will be able to give advice encompassing much more than cut-and-dried technicalities, including compassion and empathy for the patient in dealing with his deeper problems, thereby being a more effective healer.

The world urgently needs schools in which the existing and presently scattered knowledge will be brought in focus and disseminated in an effective way. What would be most important in such schools would be the "gathering" of necessary knowledge from different sources, and the exchange of such knowledge. Such a school would be without boundaries, discriminations or prejudices, and it would truly be an "Institution for Higher Learning." It would be an International School, an intense workshop of learning, run by the best people available on this planet, who will sow the seeds of transformation for a new and collective quantum jump in human consciousness. A Greek island in the Aegean Sea might just be the ideal place for such a school.

SUGGESTED RESEARCH

The many principles enunciated in the *Model* I have presented will require years of systematic research to verify. This research will have to be directed along channels relative to the ideas presented in this treatise—not accidentally or haphazardly as has been the case traditionally with research. To further such research, I would like to suggest some directions in which it might proceed with the existing technology. There are other ideas that have been expounded in this book which will have to wait longer before they can be conclusively confirmed. In any case, I feel that the research of which we are now capable should begin immediately. The research I propose is:

1. To evaluate the immune system of all patients entering hospitals before and after giving an antibiotic. A medical history with all details concerning the condition of their immune system should be kept in a computer and updated each time they undergo antibiotic treatment. In this way a profile of any deterioration of the immune system resulting from these treatments could be obtained.

2. To evaluate, in particular, the immune system of homosexuals after their first venereal disease, before starting antibiotics therapy and afterward, recording any alterations of immune system integrity after repeated treatment of such infections.

3. Epidemiological studies could be conducted to evaluate the effect of vaccination. In this *Model* it has been suggested that the explosion of multiple sclerosis is due to vaccination. Studies could be done to investigate this idea. We already know that in the countries where vaccination was unknown, multiple sclerosis was also unknown. Countries recently having introduced vaccination can be studied over time, at least two generations, for the incidence of multiple

sclerosis. I predict that multiple sclerosis will begin to appear in these countries.

4. Epidemiological studies to show clearly that the so-called degenerative diseases are an exclusive privilege of the developed countries which provide the best possible health care. I have previously alluded to the possible contention that the stress of the modern western lifestyle could be responsible for many chronic diseases. As I have also stated, I believe an examination of socialist societies, by nature far less stressful (due to a much-diminished emphasis on productivity and competition), will reveal similar chronic disease data.

5. Research to discover, as this *Model* suggests, that those most prone to contract AIDS have a specific predisposition in their genetic code.

RESOURCES

HOMEOPATHY

In many countries there are organizations which provide information and training on homeopathy. In the United States there are three organizations started to support George Vithoulkas' work:

International Foundation for Homeopathy
2366 Eastlake Avenue East, #301
Seattle, WA 98102
(206) 324-8230

This was started in 1978 by Vithoulkas, his first American student, Bill Gray, M.D., and his American assistant, Sandy Ross, Ph.D. Its goals are to:

—Educate the general public as to the principles and benefits of homeopathy
—Standardize the teaching of homeopathy in the world and to promote acceptance and teaching of homeopathy within standard medical schools
—Establish institutions in which homeopathy can be taught as a distinct medical discipline
—Raise the standards of preparation of homeopathic medicines

The International Foundation for Homeopathy offers introductory and ongoing seminars as well as an extensive post-graduate course for licensed professionals. Basic membership is $35 and includes a bi-monthly newsletter, referral list of homeopaths they have trained and discounts on tapes of seminars and other materials.

Health and Habitat
   76 Lee Street, Mill Valley, CA 94941
   (415) 383-6130
Health and Habitat was started by Sandy Ross, Ph.D.,
George Vithoulkas' American assistant. It is a 501 (c) (3)
California public benefit corporation to which donations are
tax-deductible. Its main purposes are:
   —To promote the holistic approach to life, health and the
   environment, and to help achieve a healthy state of
   equilibrium through education, research, homeopathy,
   conservation of natural resources and charity.
   —To disseminate information in the public interest concerning the above subjects through lectures, publications
   and other media.
Health and Habitat is particularly interested in promoting
homeopathy through books, videos and computer programs.

If you would like to see more material produced on the philosophy of homeopathy, case analysis, and *Materia Medicapa,*
please consider sending them a donation. H & H is the
American distributor for RADAR & THE VITHOULKAS
EXPERT SYSTEM, software which helps homeopaths prescribe correctly and successfully.

Hahnemann Medical Clinic
   828 San Pablo Avenue, Albany, CA 94706
   (510) 524-3117
The Hahnemann Medical Clinic was started by a group of
Vithoulkas' students under the direction of Dr. Roger
Morrison. It treats patients with acute and chronic diseases,
and offers a two-year training in classical homeopathy for
licensed health professionals. Associated with the clinic is the
non-profit Homeopathic Patients Foundation.

Other organizations offering information, memberships or training:

National Center for Homeopathy
801 North Fairfax Street, Suite 306
Alexandria, VA 22314
(703) 548-7790
Membership ($35), newsletter, classes for laypersons, health professional courses.

American Institute of Homeopathy
1585 Glencoe, Denver, CO 80220
(303) 321-4105
Professional organization of medical doctors and dentists; journal.

National College of Naturopathic Medicine
11231 S.E. Market Street, Portland, OR 97216
(505) 255-4860
Four-year course leading to N.D. degree, homeopathy one of the specialities, journal *Simillimum.*

John Bastyr College of Naturopathic Medicine
144 N.E. 54th Street, Seattle, WA 98105
(206) 523-9585
Four-year course leading to N.D. degree, including classes in homeopathy and acupuncture.

American Association of Naturopathic Physicians
P.O. Box 33046, Portland, Oregon 97223
(503) 255-4863

Christine Kent Agency
17216 Saticoy, Box 348, Van Nuys, CA 91406
(818) 902-1060
Distribution and promotion of materials for classical homeopathy.

Homeopathic Educational Services
2124 Kittredge Street, Berkeley, CA 94704
(510) 649-0294
Books, tapes, medicine kits, software, lectures and catalogue.

Foundation for Homeopathic Education & Research
5916 Chabot Crest, Oakland, CA 94618
(510) 649-8930
Educating professionals and the public on research and
sponsoring studies.

Kent Associates
P.O. Box 39, Fairfax, CA 94978
(415) 457-0678
MacRepertory (homeopathic software), HomeoNet

HomeoNet
Institute for Global Communications
3228 Sacramento Street, San Francisco, CA 94115
(415) 923-0900
International computer network to communicate, research,
consult and share.

Richard Pitcairn, D.V.M., Ph.D.
1283 Lincoln Street, Eugene, OR 97404
(503) 342-7665
Veterinarian practicing and conducting training programs in
homeopathy.

Liga Medicorm Homoeopathica Internationals
c/o Dean Crothers, M.D., National Vice President
23200 Edmonds Way, Edmonds, WA 98026
(206) 542-5595
International Association of physicians and scientists, journal.

The Faculty of Homoeopathy
The Royal London Homoeopathic Hospital
Great Ormond Street, London WC1N 3HR, England
Training for physicians, directory, *British Homoeopathic Journal.*

Society of Homoeopaths
2 Artizan Road
Northampton, NN1 4HU, England
Non-medical homoeopaths, directory, *The Homoeopath.*

Homoeopathic Medical Research Council
c/o The Faculty of Homoeopathy
The Royal London Homoeopathic Hospital
Great Ormond Street, London WC1N 3HR, England
Coalition of British Homoeopathic Research organizations.

British Homoeopathy Research Group
c/o Dr. Anita Davies
101 Harley Street, London W1N 1DF, England
Academic group evaluating research protocols, *Communications.*

British Homoeopathic Association
27a Devonshire Street, London W1N IRJ, England
Lay organization supporting development of homoeopathy, *Homoeopathy.*

ACUPUNCTURE

American Association of Acupuncture and Oriental Medicine
5473 - 66th Street North, St. Petersburg, Florida 33709
(813) 541-2666 or (813) 797-1161
Professional association.

National Council of Acupuncture Schools & Colleges
American City Building #100, Columbia, MD 21044
Information on where to learn acupuncture.

National Commission for the Certification of Acupuncturists
1424 16th Street, N.W., #105, Washington. D. C., 20036
(202) 232-1404
Certification based on education and testing, directory of
acupuncturists available.

Traditional Acupuncture Foundation
American City Building #100, Columbia, MD 21044
(301) 997-4888
List of Worsley classes and graduates

Quan Yin Clinic
1748 Market Street, San Francisco, CA 94102
(415) 861-4964
A non-profit organization specializing in HIV-positive patients. Certification program for treating HIV-positive patients with acupuncture and Chinese herbs.

OSTEOPATHY

American Osteopathic Association
142 East Ontario Street, Chicago, Illinois 60611
(312) 280-5800
Directory of osteopathic colleges, hospitals, and physicians
and general information about osteopathy.